AF444146

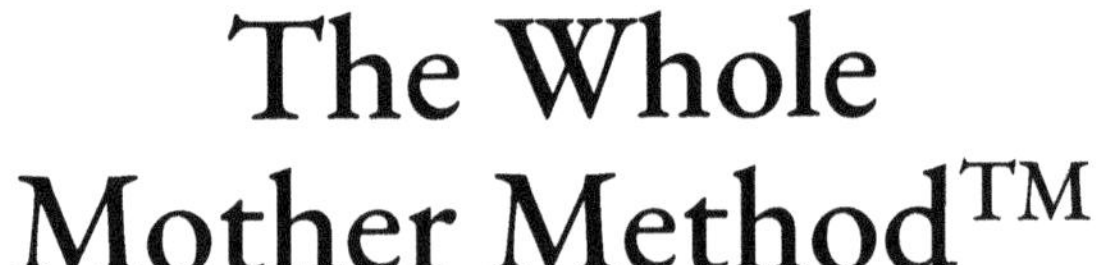

The Whole Mother Method™

How to Call Back Your Voice from the Pain of C-section Birth Trauma and Renew Your Spiritual Power

Laura Eustache Zamor, BCDN

The Resilient Writer's Project
Fleetwood, NY 10552, USA
www.llhproductionsllc.com

The Resilient Writer's Project is a division of LoLo's Light House Productions, LLC.

Published 2024

ISBN:
9798218198602

Cover Design:
Laura Eustache Zamor

Interior Formatting & Design:
Zara Danyal

Editing:
Katie Booth

Author's photo courtesy of :
Laura Eustache Zamor

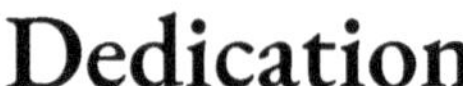

Dedication

———

To my children, you are my personal miracles. Love you always.

To my husband Kenny, for walking up morne tapion with me, and
never letting go.

To every mother in search of a voice, restored.

Table of Contents

Part I
On the Road to Getting Better

Part II
Steering Your Path to Healing

Part III
The Whole Mother Method

Conclusion

Laura Eustache Zamor

Preface

In the Christian tradition, in which I was raised, the ability to testify and witness is the ability to use the throat chakra or the voice effectively, to share about the goodness of God with others. This usually happens when you've been able to overcome a major trial, tribulation, or season of testing. You are called upon, by faith, to share with others for the edification of their growth and spiritual health. By sharing what you have managed to overcome, the telling of your story helps them to believe in the goodness of an all-encompassing God. And in this book, we are going to explore just that: how to rebuild the most precious aspect of your spiritual power as a mother—your voice.

It is not often we get a chance to see the inner workings of a mother's postpartum journey, especially what happens to her ability to practice self-advocacy around her body, and the ways in which she would like to control her path to healing after a traumatic birth. This is in part due to Western society's disregard for the sacredness of motherhood and its intense demand for adjustment to a totally new way of being and operating. An interruption or hiccup in the process is often viewed as something that should be kept private, something that should be relegated to the private spaces of counseling and therapy. Mothers are expected to have it all together, even if they are not sure how to go about that or are in search of methods that stretch beyond conventional approaches.

However, my generation of mothers, millennials, have transformed the way we discuss these aspects of our experience. With our more vocal approach—through the medium of social media and, particularly, the comments section of motherhood community pages—comes another extreme opposite from our mothers' time. This approach of sharing to be heard, to feel connected, and to stay somewhat socially active on a peer level is extreme because many of the sensitive aspects of motherhood are not being shared from a healed or self-aware perspective. The imbalances of the throat chakra are on display for all the world to see. While this might not seem like such a big deal or bad idea, the imbalance shows itself as more of a shouting match or shaming of fellow mothers who may not be walking in step with those around them. Let's highlight some examples: breastfeeding vs. bottle feeding, working mom vs. stay-at-home mom, married mom vs. single mom, crunchy mom vs. fast food mom, minimalist mom vs. fashionista mom, private mom vs. on-brand public mom—and the list can truly go on. In the case of this book and motherhood at large, is the discussion around vaginal birth vs. cesarean birth. The extreme within this grouping can be observed, again in these comments sections, as deep shaming and pushback against the mere mention of how dangerous, unfair, life-changing, and regretful the experience of having a traumatic c-section birth really is. This shaming within the walls of a me vs. you context is obviously missing what needs demystifying most: what is behind a traumatic c-section birth and some mothers' feelings around it being a less-than-stellar experience. We as women and mothers would be better advocates for each other if we used these spaces to better understand each other, rather than seeking to just be heard, a quality of a balanced throat chakra. However, because we've been on a quest to have our truth heard and accepted by society, but haven't always been successful, this imbalance is perhaps just a signaling that our individual wounds are deeper and more complex than a comments section was designed to hold. This is a book about transforming the wound from the inside out.

Here in this book, my goal is to give you permission to speak your truth, and acknowledge how hard it can be to heal from a traumatic c-section birth experience. Through the breaking down of complex body systems, emotions, and functions, along with the demystification of what really constitutes holistic healing approaches and modalities, my hope is that you are able to determine the best path towards your healing without guilt, shame, or fear. And through personal stories, that of my own journey and the amazingly resilient women I've had the pleasure of speaking with and supporting, my final hope is that you are able to anchor yourself into the practices of The Whole Mother Method: a gentle, practical, sustainable approach to putting back together the very scattered, fragmented pieces of your voice. In using this approach, may you emerge from this season of your journey vibrant, grounded, and much more nourished—mind, body, and spirit. It is my sincere belief the Creator intended motherhood to be a journey filled with boldness, power, and unwavering connection to Him. May this guide serve as a vehicle, guiding your return home to an empowered, Matriarchal self.

Author's Note

———

This book is ultimately about building back your life, and how you communicate about your life, after experiencing c-section birth trauma. We will do this through an original framework I have created, which is a culmination of original thought rooted in the experiential wisdom of my own birthing and healing process. It is informed by the traditions of yoga, specifically restorative; the philosophies and practices of traditional naturopathy; Traditional Chinese Medicine, and theories of positive psychology, specifically wellness-based. All names and events have been changed to protect the identities of others. The stories and examples used in this book are taken from clients, podcast guests, and women I have spoken with, who have given me their permission to illustrate the points made in the work through their stories. While details may have been changed to protect their identity, their core experiences and what has been shared is true.

This book is meant to serve as a companion regardless of where you are on your journey, but it may be most helpful right after having given birth, also known as early postpartum, which lasts well past the first year in some cultures outside of the Western world. Using scientific language to describe aspects of the body and how it functions, alongside traditional positive psychology, this book and its methods are grounded in tried and true clinical thought, while allowing room for the deeply personal experience of spirituality, contemplation, and self-examination. This book is part love letter to a fellow mother and part resource. Please do not substitute any part of this work for traditional therapy or medical consultation. Please note, no part of this work should be used in replacement of the care and guidance of your healthcare provider. Use your heart's discernment and use what resonates, and know that what doesn't resonate doesn't apply to your path. No part of this work should be taken as a means to diagnose, treat, or cure any illnesses of the mind, body, or spirit, nor is it written with the intent to circumvent your faith and faith-based practices. The method introduced in this book should be treated as a new idea and approach to help facilitate the restoration mothers are desperately in need of. The goal is to provide education and permission to validate your voice, your experience, and your journey to wholeness.

Introduction

——

I had hyperemesis gravidarum, a debilitating gestational condition, and after learning that my cherished obstetrician was pregnant herself and on leave, I took the advice of friends and joined a medical group's practice at a prestigious hospital. I was under the care of an all-female team and my primary caretaker was a Black woman of Ghanaian descent, whom we'll call Dr. Sarah. We struck up a good conversation because of the group's practice review but also because she was obviously a Black woman; one who had been to my family's country of Haiti and had delivered babies there, so I thought she understood the culture and the role the family of origin plays in decision making around maternal care and pregnancy. Our rapport got off to a good start, but it became clear she did not like being asked too many questions, nor did she like my husband's normal desire to be on video call during our visits since his schedule could never match up with appointments. She made it clear that she wanted to be trusted to care for me without the monitoring she perceived him to be doing. She seemed to be forgetting this was normal for a Haitian family. When present, husbands and fathers are always an active and supportive part of the expecting mother's experience. I developed pretty early on, after the HG phased, a condition called polyhydramnios and was considered high-risk almost immediately. I was told I would need to be seen weekly by specialists to observe the baby's growth in the midst of a heightened fluid state. I had one Caucasian, mid 40's OB who was also a mother and an Asian OB who were assigned to me. The baby was fine the entire time, hitting benchmarks for every measurement and evaluation. By the time I had reached about 33 weeks, I had a video call conversation with my grandmother who told me by the looks of the way I was carrying, I would not make it to the anticipated or desired 40 weeks.

Knowing our lineage and family history, I already knew it was a miracle that I had made it to a viable child number two. We had already suffered a miscarriage between these two children. I knew the women in my mother's lineage did not carry babies all the way to 40 weeks and after my experience with my first born, I wasn't scared. I knew to prepare myself. During the following visit, I took our rapport to mean I could share anything with Dr. Sarah, and proceeded to share what my grandmother had said. I was absolutely flabbergasted when she responded with how she "couldn't compete with my grandmother's bush wisdom," but that I needed to stop calling in an early labor and "pray to Jesus that we keep this baby in as long as possible. We were not delivering before 40 weeks." It was the first time in my life where I felt like my body no longer belonged to me. This situation felt different. I knew I was in trouble, but I had no idea how I was going to get out of it. When I went home and shared with my husband and family, they shared my sentiment that getting placed somewhere else under the care of someone else was going to be my best bet. Unfortunately, as I began to make calls to friends, asking about their care providers, many of them were receiving care from the same hospital. Gathering information from family friends who were nurses, I sought to get information from them about other care providers, only to learn I was too far along and too high risk to be a new patient. I was devastated, but also trying to stay calm so as not to activate a preeclamptic state.

It became increasingly clear not only the power struggle I was engaged in, but my doctor's perception of me. She wasn't looking at me as a mother who was deeply connected to her intuition and wanting to make the best decision not only for herself, but also for her baby. She was looking at me as a mother who just wanted the pregnancy to be over, which was far from the truth. I had a deep knowing that if I wasn't listened to, things would take a turn for the worst. I was just too scared to push back against her because she was Black like me and she was my doctor!

Regardless of what anyone thought, nature began demonstrating how valid my concerns were. The way I began to carry changed over the next three weeks. What was already a difficult pregnancy was becoming crippling to the point of concern with the specialists I was seeing. At 36 weeks, it was becoming increasingly difficult for me to walk or stand as the water added an additional weight to my frame. Nerve pain became a regular part of my day, as well as some difficulty breathing.

As these things started to develop, I wasn't scared, I was aware and ready to take necessary action to protect not just my baby, but myself. During my 37th week visit, the specialists agreed that having an induction by the time I reached just shy of 37 weeks and five days would be my safest bet. The Caucasian specialist told my mother and me all of the textbook information around what an induction could do to a baby's lungs, but because he was in top shape on all levels, her concern was more geared to me. She spoke very clearly about her concerns around possible hemorrhaging, rupture, and other possibly damaging early postpartum issues, resulting from the amount of water present in my womb brought on by the Polyhydramnios. She informed me that it was truly my decision as a mother and that she respected my intuition, especially as a mother herself. The only exception she mentioned was that Dr. Sarah would have to sign off on the induction for it to be performed. Upon asking her permission, she said she didn't agree, and initially refused. The power remained in her unyielding hands.

However, a week and a half after this visit, I started experiencing signs of prelabor. I knew this was the time my grandmother had talked about. He was trying to come naturally just as she said he would, but to my complete and utter shock, when we arrived at the hospital, every effort was made to stop the contractions. I was first told that I was dehydrated and all I would need was some routine IV and then I would be released to go home. However, once the nurses switched shifts, I was told my contractions wouldn't stop and I would need to take medication. I was first given Procardia- a calcium channel blocker and chest-pain focused medication. I remembered the red colored pill from my experience with preeclampsia and despite feeling in my gut that I shouldn't take it, I felt pressure from the nurse on rotation. Less than ten minutes after taking it, I was told I would need to take an injection in my leg. I began to ask questions because not only had not enough time gone by, but I was simultaneously being hooked up to another IV. As I began to ask questions, my nurse said she didn't want any problems (she was caucasian and this was when President Trump was getting ready to take office). My nurse thought I would feel better talking to the head of the medical group, a nearly 6-foot tall, Black woman who came in brazenly, saying, "I heard you don't wanna take the injection. I'm sure you don't want to be here all night. Your husband looks tired. I'm sure he wants to go home. He can, but you can stay here all night with me." The words alone raised every hair on my body. When she noticed we weren't intimidated or moved by the horrible bedside manner, she began to explain why it was her recommendation that I take the shot. She said I didn't want to run the risk of having the baby too early and that this was the "right thing" to do. With what felt like a ton of bricks on my chest and the eerie feeling they wouldn't have discharged me without taking it, I caved and took it. I was released after the IV ended, and my baby stopped moving for the next eight hours –something I would later learn was a major side effect of the medication I was given. He would never regain his normal movement in my womb.

Only after all this happened and she was fully witnessing my frame and health begin to suffer, did Dr. Sarah decide the induction was beyond necessary. But despite arriving at this conclusion, she resisted every effort to get the paperwork done to move forward with it. She went so far as to tell me the decision could not be supported because my former obstetrician never had my bloodwork and original paperwork transferred to her practice. I want you to envision being told at the final hour, after 30-something weeks of care, that your practitioner never had your paperwork and never thought to make sure it was in order.

To keep myself from going into emotional overdrive while waiting, I sought the support of a friend from undergrad who was also a doula. Miles away, on another continent, she listened to me as I lamented my deep-seated, growing fear. I wanted the baby to do what he had done before. I wanted him to leap and kick and show signs he was coming, but there was nothing. I had faith, but I was also human and developing a deeper-seated dread of the situation I found myself in.

At almost 39 weeks, I was given the date for the induction and on this scheduled night we went in. I was nervous and not at ease, but I had two amazing nurses who sought to keep me smiling and engaged every step of the way. We shared stories about our husbands and families, details about birthday parties we'd done as first-time moms and things we were most proud of as moms. As much as they tried to clear the low-hanging-cloud-like energy that seemed to be present, it was clear my doctor was angry an induction was taking place. From the way she performed the induction to the way she interacted with these nurses, the tension grew to a boiling point where she was reprimanded for yelling at one of them while I was being instructed to push. As soon as I started to push, I knew something was wrong. Having done this before, I felt it. Something was wrong. I couldn't describe what it was but I knew no matter how I positioned my breath or how much strength I gave, no progress was being made. Dr. Sarah began to insult me, telling me it was my fault because I was refusing to push. Blood came, water came just as the specialists warned, but no baby. Every time they would see his head, it would go right back up. They turned me on all fours and turned me back again. It was to the point where the pain was so intense, my eyes rolled to the back of my head, I began losing consciousness, and could feel myself leaving my body. I had heard of these outer body, near-death experiences before, but I knew this was real, and as I asked God and what appeared like an angel to take me, I was told, "No," and that "my time wasn't up yet." Then one of my nurses was smacking my leg intensely and telling me to "stay with her." As I came to, I heard the trigger-pulling words as they frantically rolled off my obstetrician's tongue, "she's not pushing properly, we need to prep the OR." I fell back onto my bed weeping, telling my husband sorry, but that something was not right. I watched the lights blur above me as I was rolled into the operating room, where an anesthesiologist greeted me. I was asked my name and if I authorized them to give me a needle along my spine. Frantically panicking, I simply begged them to make sure it wasn't an epidural. I was assured that it wasn't and after what felt like an overwhelming need to vomit while intense pressure to my abdomen was applied, I heard everyone including my husband squeal for joy as our son made it out. Turns out my maternal instincts were right. He refused to come down because he was face up or what is known as "facing forward" and was getting stuck on my pubic bone. As the obstetrician took him out, his hip wasn't pulled out properly. He was sent to the NICU immediately and we were offered no opportunity for skin-to-skin.

After three days in the hospital, and having seen everyone on the medical team, except my primary OBGYN and the OBGYN who gave me the steroid injection, Dr. Sarah walked in. I couldn't look directly at her because it felt like my heart was about to stop. As she slowly walked in, it wasn't hard to tell she was walking on eggshells. Greeted by complete silence, she motioned towards the foot of my bed and asked me how I was feeling. Not able to immediately respond, she attempted some mindless chatter before she broke into tears. Profusely apologizing, she began telling me she couldn't come to see me any faster because she was so sorry, that she had seen my son's face in her dreams since his birth, how she couldn't stop thinking about what had happened. How her greatest two fears came true: I ended up with a c-section and my son ended up in the NICU.

When she managed to finally catch her breath, tears still streaming down her face, I could only look past her shoulder at the muted television to keep from melting off of the bed—that's how mad I was. My husband, who kept his complete silence said nothing, my mother frozen in step by my bedside, everyone waiting for my reaction, she asked, "Laura, would you please forgive me? I need you to forgive me. I'm so sorry." Feeling as if the room were getting smaller by the nanosecond, I felt like I didn't know what to say. I didn't know if there was any other way out but to just forgive her. I wanted her out; I wanted to shout. I wanted to cry. I wanted it to all be over. But as if we were in a scene from one of those silent films, I simply looked at her and said, "Yes, I forgive you." I couldn't believe it came out and apparently neither could my husband because he turned around to look at me, as if to make sure he'd heard correctly and to check if I was really sure. But the truth is, I wasn't, and it wasn't until my first night home post-surgery and our follow-up visit that I would know I had given her my word prematurely. That she was just trying to get out of what I would later learn was grounds for a massive lawsuit.

I would spend the next several years of my life navigating intense change, reevaluating just what it means to incorporate rest practices in the midst of a very demanding breastfeeding journey, the rearing of a toddler, the nurturing of a young and growing marriage, and an unexpected redirecting in my vocation as a helping professional. I learned how I could trust my breath to ground me when making decisions suddenly felt like an uninvited tsunami. How I could lean into the gentle yet emotionally transformative nature of aromatherapy when feelings of rage threatened to turn my heart into stone and my words into cutting daggers. I would learn how to accept the losses that came with not returning to a professional role I loved so much, losses in personal confidence, and what felt like direction. I would learn how to use the tools of everyday life like fresh alkaline water, taking time to intentionally eat foods that bring nourishment to my physical body; respecting how much sleep I really, truly needed to function at my most optimal and not the crash-course sleep I thrived on in undergrad.

I would learn how I could redefine my sense of sensuality and sexuality after the loss of what I considered my favorite and most beautiful, but often perceived as vain quality (my hair). I would learn how I could lean into consistent journaling practices and the restructuring of a prayer life that would expose some deeply embedded roots of perfectionism stemming from the generational patterning that having children could cause you to lose everything you'd worked hard to create, professionally. I would experience the abundance of growth that would come from learning to accept lengthy seasons of intense limitation despite the influences of an outside "go-go-gadget," instant gratification culture. I would learn how, in these deep seasons of limitation and sometimes isolation, I could trust and surrender into the grace of God. I could release my grip on the notion of too much time passing and trust what this painful process was trying to teach me–where it was leading me. I could accept this season as an invitation to redirect my personal will and initiate healing in a way that felt aligned. My motherhood, and this version of entrance into this next stage of it, wasn't sent to destroy me; I was deeply loved by the Divine and I could trust the newer, kinder, more self-compassionate voice emerging from the ashes of what I once considered one of the worst experiences of my adult life.

Part I.

—

On the Road to Getting Better

Chapter 1

Gratitude as the Band-Aid

——

The first of January, in any Haitian household, is a cause for celebration. Humbly commemorating our ancestors' honorable fight for independence as the first free Black republic in the Western hemisphere, it's a time when matriarchs compete to serve the very best version of Soup Joumou, or squash soup, to their families and friends alike. Fine white china, brand new eating utensils, champagne, and freshly baked bread and patties filled with everything from herring or codfish to chicken or beef can be found across tables everywhere. In our house, a new baby and his mom had just survived a near-death c-section. With the whispers of prayers, followed by loud laughter and conversation of family members and close friends who'd come to share in the joy of both causes for celebration, I quietly sat in my silk floral pajamas and a top knot that hadn't been combed in days. Slowly sipping the soothingly creamy soup, I simply tried to take it all in.

I was just happy I could make it up the stairs to my parents' apartment without wincing. Just shy of two weeks after giving birth, there were so many things I was advised not to do and actually couldn't do. Sitting for extended periods of time, getting in and out of my bed, and even using the bathroom became acts of defiance—the pain was supernatural. Being at this family gathering, quietly taking in all the congratulations, just confirmed how different I felt this time around. Things were definitely different this time, pain being one difference, but a numbing gratitude was another. Gratitude had wrapped itself around me like a tightly woven blanket as time itself seemed to stand still. It had become my emotional Novocaine amidst the haze of figuring out what day it was or how many times I had to lay flat on my carpeted bedroom floor so my husband could both clean and redress the area around my stitching. In those moments, sheer disbelief around what I had just gone through sought to make a permanent stay, but my commitment to gratitude wouldn't allow it. "I survived!" I would tell myself. There was so much to be thankful for. "Just focus on getting through the pain. Just try to get some sleep," I'd tell myself as I tried not to concentrate on the nightmares and flashbacks that began to surface. All I knew, could focus on, and that mattered, was that I was now a mother of two boys and any time I felt the edges of shock try to pierce through, I'd double down. However, over the next two months, as these foreign experiences continued to set in, the haze of gratitude and conscious effort to double down would come to a screeching halt. And this all started one fateful Sunday morning in March.

As I sat down in one of my favorite blue terry cloth robes, I took a moment to gather myself with a soothing cup of coffee, after an early nursing session ended with the baby falling sound asleep. The sun was gently piercing the half-opened blinds of our ground floor apartment and at almost two months post-delivery, a very important conversation had taken place between my husband and me. It was a conversation most couples might face when they realize things are not going as planned or according to plan. For us, we realized that my body was not in fact healing as well or predictably as we thought it would, leading us to discuss that returning to my old position, let alone any position in student affairs, might not be the best move for me. The conversation ended with us agreeing that giving me more time, physically, was looking like the better option to proceed with. In other words: stay home. I agreed with our decision, mostly because I knew that, feeling how I was feeling, there was no way I could do any of the things I was used to doing. This surgery was beginning to change my life in ways we hadn't planned or prepared for.

The subtlety of the conversation around what was indeed becoming my new reality led me to feel several things. First off came shock, thinking things like, "I just forgave my practitioner and still had one of the worst postpartum visits a c-section mom could ever have. Like, shouldn't life be going back to normal?" I sat on the sofa feeling completely confused and, if I'm continuing in all honesty here, borderline pissed. I looked down at my very sore breasts, and an abdomen I still couldn't touch, let alone identify as my own, and suddenly realized my infinite gratitude was also masking, or dare I say suppressing, deep denial around my birthing experience. Things were not going to go back to the way they were and this moment, right here, would signal an internal shift, the trigger to opening the neatly packed emotional box of remembrance.

Granting my practitioner a verbal pardon didn't necessarily feel good, but I believed I would eventually get over everything once my life resumed its normal course of movement. I thought I was going to be okay. Reflecting on the conversation in this terry-cloth-robe moment, I realized none of this was happening and, instead, I was being forced to relinquish the normal course. All of the nicely packed anger, frustration, sense of betrayal, and resentment around how much physical pain I was actually in would begin to come rushing forth to the surface in ways I wasn't prepared for. I was waking up to the realization that my gratitude had served as a spiritual band-aid. By saying I forgave her, and doing what I thought was the spiritually astute thing to do, I thought I would be fortified to get through the physical and emotional aftermath of the near-death birth, but I wasn't. I realized I was in denial about the trauma of the delivery. And you might be too.

Because you've chosen this book, chances are you're right at the threshold of realizing the lasting impact your c-section birth is having on you and your life. You might be much further along the postpartum journey, but are just now realizing that your feelings of gratitude had long run their course of masking. Perhaps the only reason you fear acknowledging true emotional change is because you don't want to feel ashamed for not leaning deeper into gratitude, but I want you to know it's okay to acknowledge gratitude's emotional limitations. You don't have to live in denial about how the life you are returning to after this birth might look wildly different than what you anticipated, and that your actual physical and emotional pain is weighing heavier than the bliss of gratitude. You are still very much a spiritual being, but in order to accept this event's unpleasant shakeup of your life and eventually make peace with it, you're going to have to allow yourself to accept that birth trauma as a very real thing. You have to accept that c-section birth trauma, more specifically, can take its toll on your mind, body, and spirit when denied the space to be fully acknowledged.

I understand your acceptance of it may lead to the waking up of more shadow emotions like anger or rage, sadness, disappointment, resentment, or regret. I understand you might fear the sudden labeling of having a mental health issue or being labeled as possibly suffering from postpartum depression. However, the surfacing of these emotions I mentioned, manifesting as your disinterest in things like food or laughter with friends, or frustration because you can't see how household bills will get paid if you can no longer contribute, can be seen less as spiritual failure to be grateful to be alive, and more as experiencing the effects of shock and grief. With that being said, it is important to understand that there is a big difference between waking up to birth trauma, especially when it involves recovering from a major abdominal surgery, and postpartum depression. While signs might seem to overlap, one really does come before the other and if left unresolved can become the other. To make sure you're understanding what waking up to the trauma might look like and what has actually happened to the systems that make up your mental, emotional, and physical bodies, I'm going to break down each. This clarity can help you to take your first step past denial.

What is Birth Trauma?

Let's start by defining the actual term "birth trauma." While we may have heard this term shared through hashtag awareness movements on social media platforms, we seldom know how to define it or realize there are different experiences that can constitute it, causing us to engage dialogue from a place of throat chakra imbalance. By official definition, The Birth Trauma Association of the United Kingdom defines "birth trauma" as a "short-hand phrase for PTSD after childbirth." It is also used for "women who have some symptoms of PTSD, but not enough for a full diagnosis." Birth trauma or "post-natal PTSD," as it is defined by this organization, breaks identifiers down into four distinct markers:

re-experiencing the traumatic events through nightmares or flashbacks resulting in panic and distress, avoiding anything that reminds you of the traumatic event like the hospital or even songs, hypervigilance where you are irritable or constantly alert for fear something bad will happen to your baby, and finally, feelings of guilt, shame, personal responsibility, or unhappiness.

Whether it is the flashbacks that begin to surface (like they did for me) or the presence of emotions such as guilt, shame, personal responsibility, or unhappiness, by the mere definition of birth trauma, we are able to see how experiencing these emotions doesn't automatically make you a sufferer of a mental health issue. Instead, we see how the emotions are a reflection of your body being thrown into shock during one of the most emotionally transformational periods of your life: becoming a mother.

What is C-Section Birth Trauma?

While c-section birth trauma is not a clinically distinctive title, it's important to recognize the trauma that results from an emergency c-section. Both The Birth Trauma Association of the United Kingdom and The Australasian Birth Trauma Association highlight how "the many variables associated with an emergency c-section can be attributed to a mother developing post-natal PTSD." Being rushed into an operating room, and being given a spinal or epidural anesthesia, and in some cases a general anesthetic, is why 1 in 5 women develop the condition to begin with. While studies reveal what causes birth trauma for a vaginal birth, including "high levels of medical intervention, poor pain management or relief, lengthy labor, lack of dignity or privacy, past sexual abuse or violence-based trauma and harsh treatment by hospital staff members ," when it comes to c-section birth, these key factors still exist, but are compounded by a few others. These include language being used that a mother might find forceful, coercive, or simply degrading. Were you told your pushing was ineffective during labor? Did staff take the time to explain why the emergency c-section was needed or why the word "emergency" was even being used? Here, we see how the throat chakra can become unbalanced and how the events that led up to your c-section clearly set the stage for developing birth trauma or post-natal post-traumatic stress.

While we have just explored the various causes for birth trauma via vaginal births, the need for intervention via cesarean can also leave a mother feeling responsible. For example, the reasons for c-section intervention tend to involve the use of language like "labor progressing too slowly, intravenously given oxytocin is unsuccessful at stimulating more forceful uterine contractions [Merck Publications, 1467], abnormal fetal heart tracing, non reassuring fetal status or failed operative vagina delivery [Merck Publications, 1467]," or the most difficult underlying cause which can happen way before the delivery room— power struggles with practitioners that involve a mother not being listened to during labor. All of these underlying causes can leave a mother feeling guilty, shamed, responsible, weak-willed, and deeply confused about the c-section experience. When I realized how many of us might be navigating this silently, I felt called to connect through a medium that was just beginning to flourish at the time. I started the podcast, "#thebeautifulstruggle" and other women's stories started flowing towards me, stories like Sarah's and Mallory's.

Sarah's c-section delivery is a perfect example of labor not always being perceived as a purely physiological event. Wanting to give birth naturally, Sarah advocated for as much space and freedom as possible to birth naturally while laboring with her first son. She felt most comfortable walking between and through the contractions. However, after being told by staff that she needed to labor on her back rather than deliver standing as she and her husband had advocated for, progress became stalled. She was told by doctors the head of her child could be seen but movement was stalled. Sarah was then told she needed to have an emergency c-section. As she was being told these details, Sarah could feel her spirit tank with the heaviness of this birthing intervention not being what she truly wanted. She immediately felt the flood of fear and confusion, as memories of her mother's emergency c-section story immediately came to mind. Sarah's mother flatlined during her c-section surgery and this became an immediate fear for

[1] Soderquist, J., Wijma, K., & Wijma, B. Traumatic Stress after Childbirth: The Role of Obstetric Variables. Journal of Psychosomatic Obstetrics & Gynecology, (2002) 23(1), 31–39.

[2] Kim Thomas, "What is Birth Trauma?" The Birth Trauma Association, 2018, https://birthtraumaassociation.org.uk/for-parents/what-is-birth-trauma.

Sarah. Not having control over the direction of the delivery and being told the only way to progress was through c-section delivery led her to feel extremely sad. Another example of mothers who feel responsible for the need to deliver via cesarean, is Mallory's story.

Mallory's* Story

As an executive who worked long hours, Mallory was most concerned with the state of an opening cervix throughout her third pregnancy. Mallory began bleeding prematurely and was forced to deliver via c-section earlier than 25 weeks gestation. She bore the feelings of responsibility and what she describes as early stages of depression after watching her newborn on life support for several months. Not only was she dealing with the shock of what her body had gone through ahead of scheduled time, she carried the emotional labor of waiting for her daughter to completely heal. Mallory's experience isn't necessarily about power struggle or coercion, yet it is a classic example of how a mother can struggle to find her testimony around a birth because so many factors seemed to reinforce her shame around how the birth ended up being cesarean. She had feelings of confusion and remorse and felt like she could have prevented this from happening by getting more rest.

Each of these stories demonstrate the complex nature of what causes c-section birth trauma and why it can be difficult to move forward. Like these mothers, and many others whose names we don't know, putting back the pieces of her life can become stunted by shame taking over and silencing even the ability to talk about the fact that you have a lack of gratitude over surviving the birth. This can also signal why, for some mothers, it can take years to feel better or cultivate a healthier version of self where personal expression around the experience is one of acceptance, surrender, and peace. Instead, this silent battle of shame and fear around revealing signs of post-traumatic, postnatal stress can manifest as the actual development of deep depression or things like thyroid imbalances, constant sore throats, either speaking too loudly or too softly, gastrointestinal discomforts or altogether shying away from speaking. These are the long-term telltale signs that a mother hasn't given herself the space to accept how gratitude can indeed act as a tool for denying the presence of c-section birth trauma.

In order to experience the freedom of healing, and choose to activate this in a holistic way, it is important to understand how your entire system is impacted by this type of experience. Understanding your body and how it is responding to what has happened to it is key to navigating the surefooted emotions that can take over once the goo goo gaga stage of newborn life fades. While there are 11 systems in total that make up the human body, for the purpose of this book, we are going to focus on what I believe are the three most important to calling your voice back from c-section birth trauma and being able to fully restore your spiritual power. These systems are the Nervous system, the Digestive system, and the Endocrine system. The entire method is built around supporting these three major orchestrations of the body and you will hear me reference them throughout, so let's get acquainted with how they are actually impacted.

The Nervous System

We have to remember that every part of us is connected. From organs and blood, to emotions and thoughts. I believe our bodies were a physical creation to demonstrate creative expression and in this same vein, once I had the c-section, it made me wonder why birth and postpartum were not central parts of our learning experience while in high school or even in college. I don't know about you, but all I could remember was the very mechanical explanation of fertilization, pregnancy and a baby coming out of the vagina. I do not remember even the slightest mention as to what the process, let alone the types of birth, does to the body as a whole—mind, body, or spirit. There was never any conversation, not even in the realms of personal-social-emotional development curriculum around who or what the mother becomes as a result of her birth or the early stages thereafter. As a member of middle sec Gen-Y, sexual education consisted of extremely mechanical terms with a focus of just "getting through" the material. However, as a Catholic, all-girl school graduate, I would have appreciated the focus on motherhood, from not so much a perspective of fear so as not to get into it before my time, but a focus on the intensity and complication that pregnancy and delivery truly are as an experience. This presentation of truth and education would have perhaps saved an entire generation from having to look for viable childbirth education via social media. Something else I would have appreciated, and maybe you too, would have been exposure to what changes happen to the mind and spirit as a woman steps onto the entirely new plane of motherhood, as this plane is such an important fabric of life and literally sustains society. Indeed, we know healthy mothers make for healthy societies.

Now if you are among the mothers who did invest in books, classes, and sessions to prepare for birth, non-influenced by social media, were you prompted to pick up books on both natural births and cesarean births? For me, the answer was a resounding, "No!" Not until preparing for a three-part series for my podcast in 2020 did I truly investigate what books have to say about the effects of a cesarean birth, in particular. I learned a few things rather quickly. Firstly, much of what we are taught, as women of a certain age, is how our bodies are these overly intricate things whose functioning can only be entrusted to those in the allopathic medical field. There is a mechanical approach to healing time frames, where there is no mention of how it can take almost a whole year to regain sensation from the abdomen incision. The second thing I learned from my inquiry is how our mind, body, and spirit do not function interchangeably, but rather separate; any signs of negative emotional reaction is automatically a sign of mental illness rather than being perceived as the body expressing distress, which can manifest as anger, disappointment, or even rage about what led to the surgery to begin with. Not only was this perspective of mind-body unification not included in the books I was prompted to read, but mention of the spirit was nowhere to be found. While there was clinical mention of therapists and counselors to seek out, should symptoms of postpartum depression surface, there was no alert to how your faith and spiritual life might be impacted. There was no mention of how feeling disconnected from, or even abandoned by, Source could be a contributing factor to never feeling like things could be better or sense could be made of the experience.

If it has taken you longer than you expected or you were told to move beyond the physical pains of your c-section and the birth trauma that accompanied it, please take heart. A lot has happened to you and I want to teach you about how much the physical body is related to your emotions and spiritual progress. Despite what we have heard conventionally about healing and recovery, there is a mind-body and even spirit connection. Too often we are taught that when we start to experience heavy emotions, and ones that are taking some time to leave us, it's all about our brains or perhaps just hormonal imbalance—almost like the brain is this isolated organ, disconnected from the energy of the rest of the body. But how can that be? With this first system, our Nervous system, we can immediately see the interconnectedness. Separated into three parts, you might have heard about the central nervous system which encompasses the brain and the spinal cord, while our peripheral nervous system is the constitution of nerves of the body that extend from the spinal cord (31 pairs) and 12 pairs of nerves from the brain. The third part, called the autonomic nervous system, is the connection from the peripheral I just mentioned, to every organ in our bodies, sending messages to and from our brain to our organs via something called neurotransmitters which behave something like an information highway. This subsystem of the greater overall nervous system is even further divided into another subsystem called your sympathetic and parasympathetic nervous system, and both are controlled by, you guessed it, emotion. And in a very intelligent, interconnected way, in your brain beneath four distinct lobes, you have something called the limbic system. This part of the nervous system, which governs the experience and expression of emotions, stores memory and plays a chief role in mood response. Made up of various parts of such as the hippocampus, amygdala, septal nuclei, and olfactory area, which impacts smell and mood, this area of the brain and nervous system also houses the hypothalamus. The hypothalamus is the master of all master glands in the body and acts as a switch director. Based on external influences such as environments of stress or joy on the body, it sends signals to the secondary master of all secretion functions of the body, the pituitary gland. When the body is in a relaxed and agreeable state (in the case of this book, after a happy and fulfilled birthing experience) the autonomic nervous system is in a state of "rest and digest," or what they call parasympathetic. In this state, all of your organs are in a much more calmed state, your heart rate is slowed down, the muscles of your digestive tract are relaxed-and are able to manage their responsibilities because they are receiving clear guidance from these master control centers. This is in part because in the opposite state or sympathetic, you're in fight or flight mode which causes your heart rate to pick up and the parts of the limbic system register the memory of the event as one that produced fear. When you are in the middle of what seems to be a labor that is failing or rapidly changing from progressed (vaginally) to distressed or what your OBGYN might feel to be stalled and you're now faced with making a split-second decision about having major abdominal surgery, your entire system picks up on that experience. Your sympathetic nervous system is kicked into gear because hearing that your baby is in danger leads to you automatically wanting to flee that dangerous situation. Combine that with pressure to make a decision by those in charge of the experience and seem to have more knowledge than you or have simply gained your trust to do so, you're no longer making a decision in a calm, grounded mental and emotional space—and the body remembers.

Examining the birth stories of the mothers I just shared and perhaps examining your own, we are able to make the connection between why the body as a whole goes into shock: the brain gives a lot of attention to the memory of the surgery itself, as well as all the events that led up to it, creating the space for what we now know as post traumatic stress. Your limbic system is locked in the loop of replaying the event, and certain sounds, smells, or sights act as initiating triggers.

This is what is happening in the brain, to the nervous system, but what about the other systems? The other organs that make up the other ten systems of the body? How are they impacted? Surgery is over and the danger seems to have ended because you and your baby have survived. However, what has happened to the organs involved with what just transpired? What's the dialogue now happening between your adrenals, liver, lungs, heart, large intestine and the brain? Not only on the physical level but also the spiritual level? This is what we're going to explore in order to understand why it has been so difficult to relinquish feelings of not just sadness, but also betrayal, anger, vexation, self-blame, and feeling that you would have responded differently had your body been in a calmed manner. And most importantly, I will help you to understand why it might feel like you don't really have the luxury of time, but instead are given subliminal messages that rushing through the emotional discomfort of such a tragic experience is the right thing to do, that if you aren't masking these very real emotions and the changes you must be heading on a turn for the worst. We're going to explore emotions not just as feelings that influence an outward social experience, but as the energy of our birthing experiences, which circulate within the energetic meridians of the body, as well as why emotions are so crucial to healing to address the trauma of mind, body, and spirit. These experiences, when unchecked via the breaths you forget to take (REST), the inflammatory foods you are told it's okay to continue to eat as you physically heal (REPLENISH), and the confusion about how to navigate roles and responsibilities before the surgery surges forward now that time is passing (REEVALUATE), continue to circulate as blocked qi within your liver meridian, your large intestine meridian, your heart, and other vital organs. For example, according to Traditional Chinese Medicine, your liver carries the emotional energy of frustration and anger, and when not appropriately expressed, the liver can suffer from qi stagnation. Let's explore this a little deeper, as we move on to the digestive system and see how it's impacted by the experience of a traumatic c-section birth.

The Digestive System

While gratitude can be considered an expression or virtue of the heart, the organs that make up your digestive tract also have emotional consciousness that is expressed in response to what our external environment presents us with. Just like the hypothalamus releases oxytocin when you're giving birth, according to the principles of Traditional Chinese Medicine, the organs of the body are related to the types of emotional responses we have to a situation- and whether or not we can actually digest the situation itself. But in order to make the connection to what those emotions are and their corresponding organ, we have to understand how both the peripheral and autonomic nervous systems impact digestion. The autonomic nervous system controls your involuntary activity and in digestion this means swallowing and the food being pushed down your throat. The peripheral nervous system division into sympathetic state and parasympathetic state affects digestion. When you are in a sympathetic state (usually caused by something causing stress to the body, like c-section surgery, which itself is traumatic on the body) the food you take in to nourish yourself cannot do its job because the digestive process is slowed. It is not uncommon to find your appetite is cut when you are stuck in a mental loop of reliving the memories from the birth. The role and responsibility of food is to first keep you alive and second bring energy, nutrition, and vitality to your body. This includes the parts of your brain communicating back and forth with your gut via the vagus nerve. The food you are consuming during this period of recovery, as you navigate emotional responses to the birth, can do things like either calm or accelerate your heart rate, a direct result of either divisions of the autonomic system being in activation. So when conventional approaches tell you it's totally okay to "eat whatever" right after birth, we can see how drinking soda, other highly processed drinks, consuming high quantities of sugar, and fried or refined foods can actually cause more aggravation to the entire system, including more inflammation, which isn't good for gut healing post-surgery. These factors, again, impact mood as the presence of more sugar in the body can cause excitability where there is already anxiousness; more saturated fat, low fiber foods can impact circulation, causing a decrease in energy leading to fatigue.

While we have learned how postpartum depression is a collection of symptoms related to the severe, persistent mood changes a mother can experience after birth, it's not hard to see why post traumatic stress can easily be confused with postpartum depression. When you are not eating in a way that supports a healthy digestive system, it is easier for the manifestations of post traumatic stress to remain, and the prolonged sadness, loss of appetite from ruminating thoughts and the replaying of events, and signs of anger as you work to navigate a new reality can be perceived as you being headed in that depressive direction. Just know there is nothing to be ashamed of because it takes time to digest a traumatic experience, much less a traumatic abdominal birth. Experiencing sadness (beyond the sixth week, post-op), anger, disappointment, or other aspects of post traumatic stress are a pretty normal response given what we have just explored and learned here.

While having gratitude for being alive is surely an antidote to the bitter sadness of it all, it would be beneficial to give ourselves the permission to fully see ourselves while we come to have a better understanding of the vessels we've been given by our Creator. This is ultimately a holistic approach that at its core supports us becoming fully healed and not just "well enough to function." This holistic, personalized approach can also be the difference between being told to simply take a stool softener every time you feel constipated post-op (where constipation absolutely impacts mood) versus being supported on the best type of fiber to consume to help regulate your digestive tract. And in speaking of digesting your experience, the literal digestive tract itself and how food works to provide nourishment, let's continue with understanding just how this part of our vessel works in relation to your postpartum healing and recovery!

The Digestive System: How nutrients travel through the body

Beginning in the mouth, the digestive system is more than just the stomach that receives food or the colon we often hear needs cleansing. The digestive system is made up of organs that not only impact our physical health, but our emotional health as well. These organs include ones that are also considered part of the endocrine family, due to their communication of hormone regulation, and are as follows: the tongue, stomach, liver, gallbladder, small intestine, large intestine, spleen, and pancreas. The pancreas is both an exocrine and endocrine gland. In the portion of the method called Replenish, we'll make the connection even further between how what you put in your body impacts not just your physical self, but these different systems that impact emotional health as well, since everything is so delicately interconnected.

Focusing on eating whole, fresh, nourishing foods is an excellent, yet overlooked, way to support the reduction of post traumatic stress on the body. In our culture we think of food in extremes, either to be indulged or to be used for dieting, which for women is always linked to body image rather than healthfulness. We are rarely exposed to how eating nourishingly can have a massively positive impact on our emotional and spiritual bodies. This happens because when we eat nutrient dense foods, the tissues of the body receive the nutrients needed to reduce things like inflammation post-op (which when unknowingly begins to run rampant, hampers mood and emotional stability). Through the small and large intestines, respectively, the digestive system sends these nutrients to your nervous system to support the energy, and repair the body needs to function. Post a traumatic c-section birth, this is even more important. This can help to make sense of why, when you drink the right amount of fresh water daily, you're more apt to be calm and understand incoming information than when you're dehydrated. The digestive system interacts with the endocrine system as hormones secreted by the endocrine system stimulate the juices of the liver, gallbladder, and pancreas. Vitamins and minerals consumed via whole foods and absorbed through digestion in turn support healthy hormonal production, keeping the endocrine system balanced as well. This is incredibly important when considering the practice of nourishment as a means to diminish manifestations of post traumatic stress rather than exacerbate them. Here are some examples of how emotions related to post traumatic stress can be looked at in relation to the different organs of the body, which can help us to stop looking at them so separately.

Anger & the Liver: The emotion begins to show up as effects of the birth surface through unexpected routine or functionality changes. You cannot expand as you used to, which is the energy governed by the Liver.

Anger, an emotion we are taught to fear because channeled inappropriately it can lead to acts of violence, manifests as a result of feeling unable to appropriately expand. Think of a balloon that is supposed to get blown up to a healthy size without popping. Well in the context of recovering from a birth that is impeding you from creating succinct routines, or simply moving forward in what you feel is a timely manner, your liver is the organ connected to and is energetically registering this frustration. In Traditional Chinese Medicine, you are building an excess of wood energy, the liver's element, which begins to create an overall imbalance to the rest of your system. While emotionally this can look like having unexpected shouting matches with others in your home, snappy or short communication through mediums like texting or email, or even shutting down completely from feelings of others no longer understanding your effort, there are things happening on a physical level as well.

The liver, a very important player in your digestive system and largest organ in the body, is responsible for over 500 functions in your body, including the detoxification of toxins in the body; the storing of vitamins such as vitamins A, D, and K; and of course, manufacturing bile, which carries away waste, while breaking down fats during digestion. When excessive wood from emotional upsets builds in the liver, you may experience things like headaches, migraines, reddened face, or an increase in thirst. If you stick your tongue out you might even notice demarcation around the edges of your tongue.

Perfectionism & the Large Intestine: The emotion begins to show up when there's a lack of control around getting things done. Your ability to handle tasks before and after the birth has shifted and you strive to overcompensate.

An emotional response to the internal fear of failure or being harshly judged, perfectionism may manifest itself as trying to keep all your schedules intact the way you used to prior to becoming a mom. There may be a routine of prayer or how you handled groceries that simply no longer works for you, but you work ten times harder to try and make it work. Because trauma activates the amygdala, fear can become an emotion that blocks you from feeling like you can eventually get things right or that you can safely change directions entirely. Because you are healing and changes are happening in your day-to-day life, this unmitigated fear can be a signal that you are still operating from a place of fight or flight.

Hypervigilance & the Spleen: This begins to show up as you ruminate and either replay every aspect of moments leading up to the birth or constantly overthink everything you are doing to the point of obsession.

A sac-shaped organ considered both an endo and exocrine gland, the spleen is a major power player when it comes to how we process thoughts. Responsible for the circulation of healthy red blood cells and removal of destroyed ones, the spleen also governs the transformation of food and fluid we take in, as well as the production of the immune system's lymphocytes. When the spleen is physiologically strong, it runs these processes very well and we experience healthy digestion, meaning no belching, bloating, or even runny stools. However, when the spleen is weak, we can experience the opposite, including loss of appetite, restless sleep, and even palpitations. According to Traditional Chinese Medicine, the physiological functioning of the spleen becomes weakened under the emotional weight of obsessiveness, loop-like thoughts, worry, and anxiousness, directly connected to the limbic system.

The Endocrine System

Where the nervous system is what I would call the communications highway of the body, the endocrine system is what supports communication between this highway and some very important glands within your body. Specifically for us women, something like the event of birth impacts the functioning of the endocrine system. Due to this system's regulation of hormones produced by the pituitary, much of its functioning has influence over our mood. Made up of glands and organs such as the pituitary, pineal, hypothalamus, thymus, thyroid and parathyroid, adrenals, and ovaries, this system produces hormones that impact things like our ability to produce milk, have vaginal lubrication, and have uterine contractions. When you are healing from a traumatic c-section birth, the stress on your nervous system has a direct impact on the signals being sent between these glands and the pituitary gland in the brain. The signals can become distorted or off-balance depending on how much physical or emotional pain you're in. For example, epinephrine or adrenaline released by the adrenal glands can speed up your heart rate and make you feel very anxious. Perceived fear in the system and an overproduction of adrenaline now keeps your body in a sympathetic state, causing your appetite to become depleted or your stomach to hurt anytime you try to eat. This can also show up as the pineal gland no longer being able to send the proper signal for sleep and the entire circadian rhythm getting thrown off balance.

The endocrine system could be considered an especially important point of focus for us as mothers because here is where we are able to make the connection between much of the chemical function of the body, via hormones, and our electrical, energetic nature via our chakra health. While much of Western medicine has focused most strictly on the brain when it comes to addressing emotional trauma, and rightfully so as we have just explored the importance of the limbic system, the endocrine system provides connection to our chakra health. Our chakra health, explored further in the Reevaluate portion of The Whole Mother Method, bridges the connection between our physical and subtle body energy.

Our subtle body energy, through seven centers or chakras of the body, accounts for tying together everything we see, feel, and experience–within ourselves and with our external environment. These chakras also represent different aspects of our spiritual consciousness or what some might call virtues. Linked to each endocrine gland as well as your nervous system's nexus points, we can see how an emotionally disruptive birth can create imbalances not just in the brain, but the rest of the body as well. For example, the throat chakra, which governs our spiritual ability to speak our truth and to speak with integrity, is directly related to our thyroid health. If a mother were to say there is no need for c-section birth trauma to be recognized when internally she felt

[3] Pablo Noriega, Bach Flower Essences and Chinese Medicine(Healing Arts Press, 2016).

otherwise, this subtle body energy center picks up on this misalignment and can create blockages which we could externally observe as physical discomforts like hair loss or fluctuating weight. Another example is the physical health of our ovaries, which is an endocrine organ but is also directly related to the balance or imbalance of our sacral, or second chakra vibration. A mother who is not fully acknowledging that she has experienced a violation during her emergency c-section birth can experience painful periods or find it difficult to have vaginal lubrication during sex. This is why it can be extremely beneficial for us to look at our spiritual consciousness through the lens of our endocrine system as a means for healing. We can also observe how this impacts the pace at which we heal which for every mother is indeed unique.

Through highlighting the workings of each system that constitutes The Whole Mother Method and how they've been impacted by c-section birth trauma, we can see that there is foundation for a unique relationship between how we breathe, what we eat, and how we manage our chakra energies. This unique relationship, when acknowledged, can serve to bring us back into full health at a gradual, individual pace. When acknowledged, the spiritual power of speaking our truth with integrity can be more authentically reclaimed. Our narrative around who we are, what we've experienced, and how we feel as a result of experiencing c-section birth trauma can both be acknowledged and begin to shift.

[4] Cyndi Dale, The Subtle Body: An Encyclopedia of Your Energetic Anatomy, (Sounds True, 2009)

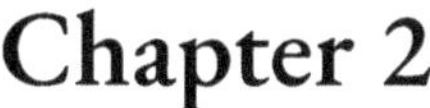

Chapter 2

Social Media & the Unsafe Comment Section

———

"Many obstetricians feel inherently that vaginal delivery is just plain dangerous, leading to increased fetal trauma. I've been in discussions with male and female colleagues who believe on some very deep, unexamined level that abdominal delivery is the superior mode of arrival. Recently some are strongly advocating elective cesareans as a matter of preference. Unfortunately, you have to be quite resilient and self-assured to resist the environment of inductions and planned C-sections that is now common in far too many hospitals."- (Christiane Northrup, M.D., "Women's Wisdom, Women's Bodies)

In the years since my birth, the presence of motherhood, birth, and postpartum education present on social media has gained massive growth and attention. One networking app in particular has become the breeding ground of mothers using their motherhood to survive, well, motherhood. And while I do not want this to read as a dig to mothers who are active with platforms earning income or providing advocacy, this newly developed need to be "on," can be disconcerting for the mother who has just experienced a traumatic c-section birth. I am especially speaking to the mom who might be feeling isolated and feeling like the best way to stay connected to others is to engage in what can sometimes be very antagonistic dialogue.

I remember when my son was first born and simply having excitement to hit send on a picture to let others know we had safely made it- that he was finally here. I also remember mustering the courage to hit "publish" on a video announcement about my podcast, inspired by the birth, but nothing compares to the present and what I have observed mothers navigating in these spaces so many years later. Years later, the excitement to share is still there, but is also marked by the need to appear as if nothing is wrong, everything is perfect, and the constant participation must still go on. There is now a present urgency that seems very much connected to the presence of managing one's personal brand, a concept that seems to have replaced my generation's understanding of public reputation. The difference is maintaining your reputation never used to involve constant personal documentation for public consumption, especially when navigating birth and motherhood. Mothers who participate in the online space for whatever reason, now with this personal brand messaging being enforced, must effortlessly glide into the often chaotic spaces of the newly post partum life with minimal interruption; no time for true downtime.

It's either that seemingly effortless perfection or the complete opposite where moms now seem to be succumbing to an undeniable pressure- perhaps again personal branding messages- to share every utter gorey aspect of those early post-birth moments, such as sharing pictures of c-section stitching and scars or saturated post-op underwear. And while this type of sharing can definitely be seen as our generation bringing a greater awareness to the often unacknowledged and stressful parts of motherhood, it is also concerning, how the need to document these moments is also taking away from the internal and external adjustment needed to experience a balanced start to postpartum. This is especially true for mothers like you, who are reading this book, who have just experienced something so transformative as c-section birth trauma.

This is not at all to say that coming together in a virtual community to talk about the very real struggles around motherhood or healing after a traumatic birth is a bad thing. It's not at all lost on me that newfound motherhood can be extremely isolating and that posting or sharing can be a way to stay connected. However, what I am saying based on tons of observation is when it comes to discussing something as tender and hot-button as c-section surgery, the lines for friendly communing and the beginnings of shaming, attempts at silencing, and maybe even mob- discrediting, quickly become blurred. At the time of my writing this book, the comments sections of social media pages are not yet a common means or methodology for gathering qualitative research on their effects on adult mental health. However, should it ever, I would not be the least bit surprised, as here in these comments sections is where one can literally gather consensus around how women discuss birth, specifically c-section birth. Here in these comments sections is where people gather to debate, but unfortunately with no real moderator present, except for the deletion or limiting of commentary by the account owner. This leaves discussion around what is considered a good birth or satisfying birth open to turning into a shouting match which in essence eats away at the larger goal of allowing us to share our experiences or learn how to support one another outside of the realms of this virtual reality. If we're going to focus on our collective healing as mothers, knowing in essence every birth story matters, we're going to need to address the ways in which social media, while recovering from c-section birth trauma, acts as the second yet major speed bump on the road to getting better.

1: Stirring anxiety and personal doubt about your experience

Many women are unaware of the complications that can arise from emergency c-sections. Unfortunately, in our Western culture, it takes certain celebrities to bring national attention to what can happen when there is insufficient post-op care, when pain isn't being properly acknowledged, or when blood clots and infections develop from c-section surgery. It's incredulous, I know, but only then are we able to see empathy or compassion extended towards those who are left navigating some very painful post-op realities. Only then, does it seem less problematic to express one's disdain with not having been able to birth vaginally. And only then, does it seem safe to step out and discuss certain complications, like poor hospital staff and environments, systemic racism within the walls of where they're giving birth, or worse, power dynamics. As a mother who might not have any type of notoriety, celebrity, or notable personal branding to speak of, trying to explain to others your point of view on the emotional trauma that emergency c-section births or unwanted c-section births can bring about, can prove to be futile. Trying to convince strangers on the internet that your trauma was perhaps totally preventable, or why mothers should ask more questions of their providers, can also prove to be tiresome. When working on activating your system's innate ability to heal itself, this is not exactly the direction you want to set your sails in.

It's not at all that you are wrong for wanting to bring what might feel like counter-awareness around c-section birth to spaces that encourage advocacy. However, within a culture and system that so often promotes division, mob-mentality approaches, and truths being targeted as misinformation, you may just be treading grounds for stirring anxiety or personal doubt around the validity of your story and contribution when trying to share. And with catch phrases like "Strong as a Mother" intended to empower the woman who perhaps did elect for a c-section delivery, you may find yourself feeling quieted or being discredited as having anti-empowerment sentiments. Turning inward and focusing on your own healing, is the first step to contributing to the healing of the feminine. By steering clear of the comments sections, even if just for a little while, you're not quitting, you're shifting.

2: Further disruption of energetic qi

For starters, when we talk about the energetic disruption traumatic experiences cause and how post traumatic stress can be experienced, we're talking about a few things. From a naturopathic perspective, as we talked about in chapter one, the meridians of the body experience a sort of backlog as the body, in its intelligence, recognizes something has brought it under shock. In this state of shock, unless you are engaged in modalities to get the qi moving again, this disruption can inhibit the system from processing the experience and letting it go. When the limbic system and the body's meridians are unable to process or release a traumatic birth, they're caught in a loop around the event marked by danger or shock. When you engage in a commentary on social media, for example through awareness month dialogues or discussions linked to magazine articles, being triggered from needing to somehow prove just how dangerous, stressful, or life-altering your experience was, weakens your vital force.

As a matter of fact, these types of exchanges only further disrupt the liver meridian because anger or resentment from being misunderstood, dismissed, or constantly tagged for a continual response, is now being stirred. Remember, your liver is where the body processes the emotions of anger and frustration, and there cannot be anything quite as frustrating as trying to express to folks whom you presume will understand, but seem to resist, just what your journey has looked like. From the research I conducted for my own podcast series on the history, uses, and overuses of c-section as a birthing intervention, I came to learn how much women have been groomed to believe the notion that c-section birth is indeed more safe than vaginal birth in some instances, leading some to hold very tightly to believing they would be dead without it. Trying to counter these deeply ingrained beliefs would be burdening your spleen meridian, which we've discussed governs rumination, being overstimulated with thinking about how to respond or preparing a response that adequately justifies your position or communicates your pain. It can honestly become obsessive, something characteristic of a depleted spleen meridian which you don't want if the main expression of your birth trauma is feelings of anxiousness.

3: Seeking Camaraderie Around a Mutual Cause

I completely understand the society we're currently living in and the way it can seem so harmless wanting to share your own experience, participate in a dialogue that might potentially save another woman's life, or even bring awareness to types of experiences other family members might need closure around; that coming together virtually around a common cause, hashtag, organization, or discussion can create a sense of social connectedness- camaraderie if you will. I know of many women who have shared making meaningful connections with other women they would have otherwise never met if not for showing up in certain spaces. This is where we see the positivity and purposefulness behind using networking apps. However, it's important to consider the very same flipside of this virtual coin. There are some who may arrive to these social media spaces ready to engage, but not always having worked through the grief of their own narratives around something like needing or even electing for a c-section birth. Getting into heated debates in the comments sections not only creates further disruption of your qi, what I mentioned above, but constant interactions of the like, during such a sensitive time of your healing journey, can undermine your desire to feel seen, heard, or understood within a group or social context. And it's not that your sentiments around the pain left behind by c-section trauma don't deserve to be heard, because they do. In fact, simply by reading this book, know that you are seen, heard, and held, and that living in this digital age might make you feel like you need to rush to participate and share, but you don't have to.

Trying to form connections, particularly as women, in a space and within a culture where we are constantly seeking to have our viewpoints heard, but can often get pitted against each other, talking about our feelings around traumatic births can become complicated when there is failure to consider issues around socioeconomic, racial, and even ethical issues that arise for women in hospitals. These issues may be very difficult to digest on social media, as these spaces very much blur the lines between fantasy and reality. Even when hashtags and movements are formed, there will still be women who may never understand the nature of power, racial, and intellectual dynamics at play when it comes to how some mothers come to experience c-section birth trauma, and even post-op complications. Here in the West, there are deeply rooted issues around the bodily autonomy of Black women, in particular. According to author Dorothy Roberts, enslaved mothers were considered simply as "breeders." In her chapter, entitled Reproduction in Bondage, she describes the plantation mentality around pain, birth and a Black mother being seen as disposable, with only the infant being a necessary commodity worth preserving. Roberts highlights for us the roots of the generational psychological stain around voice, shame, lack of autonomy, and generalized fear when engaging with practitioners. "Feminists use the term "maternal-fetal conflict" to describe the way in which law, social policies, and medical practice sometimes treat a pregnant woman's interest in opposition to those of the fetus she is carrying [Roberts, 40]. "The miracles of modern medicine, for example, that empower doctors to treat the fetus apart from the pregnant woman make it possible to imagine a contradiction between the two....Pitting the mother's interests against those of the fetus, in turn, gives the government a reason to restrict the autonomy of pregnant women [Roberts, 40].

Without direct experience in these often belittling, dehumanizing and not-so-subtle threatening power dynamics within some birthing spaces, mothers in defense of c-section birth, will not understand why you feel the need to refute the narrative that it's a "normal, safe, and should be respected life-saving intervention." In fact, some mothers who may have elected for a c-section due to their own fears around giving birth vaginally, may receive your expression as shaming them for their decisions. This can elicit responses of fear that come across as shouting back and forth in defense. By fear, I mean some mothers don't want to lose the empowerment that can be felt from the power of choice and being free to choose birth by c-section even though research shows how dangerous it can be with post-op issues around hemorrhaging, blood clots, infection, and the need to take medications our bodies might not take well to. It will be incredibly important to heal the gaping wound of generational jealousy, misinformation, and mob-mentality instead of censoring words that truly express experiences with power struggles and disappointment.

If we are sharing these experiences publicly for awareness and camaraderie, it will be incredibly important that we stop the undermining of stories and experiences of those brushed off to the side as not the majority. Instead, we should work to come to an understanding that fear drives people to do certain things while shame prevents others from doing others. More importantly, the feelings of safety, autonomy, respect, and collaboration matter to all of us. Not having received or experienced that during your birthing experience doesn't need to be debated. You do not have to use this time to prop or position yourself in a virtual space to try to bring validation to a birthing experience that maybe didn't even need to happen. Instead, you can make the personal decision to turn inward as you navigate the newest stages of your postpartum journey.

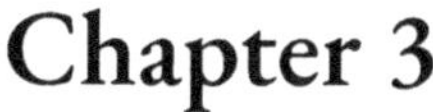

Chapter 3

The Shame of Not Suing

———

I was sitting in the kitchen with a family member from my husband's side, gently spinning on one of the stools when my birth story became the topic of conversation. I got to explaining what happened and why it is so difficult for some women, especially Black women, to trust new physicians after such a traumatic experience has happened. I was blown away by his response as he swiftly put the juice back in the fridge. "Man, that was y'alls fault. You didn't report that doctor for malpractice. You should have just sued. Simple."

I felt like I'd gotten shot in the foot or something. I felt the heat of my blood shoot to my feet then icily rise back to my head. I thought I was going to explode. But instead, I sat glued to the stool and felt a bolt of shame begin to circulate. I couldn't believe my ears. "Why didn't I just sue, asshole?" That's what I really wanted to say, but remembering where I was and how loving his mother and father had been to me, I tried to keep my composure. I responded by telling him that money couldn't do a single thing to take away all the stress, sadness, fear, and change ushered into my life simply because a physician thought she could play God on earth. Moreover, I had trusted her and pathetically told her I had forgiven her because this woman was in fact a Black woman, of African descent, just like me. Although I had been deeply violated, I was more concerned that I would be going back on my word, and for me, my word was everything. He looked at me, and again, he just uttered, "Nah, man, that was a lawsuit. Y'all coulda just pursued that."

Money doesn't solve every problem. There, I said it, and whether or not others agree, if this is how you also secretly feel, this is an opportunity to breathe a sigh of relief. That sigh comes from us both knowing how here in the West, this sentiment is not universally shared. In the society we live in, it is basically pitched to us through our favorite drama series that suing is indeed the fix-all for offenses. Here, there is a deeply ingrained belief that getting a lump sum of cash can somehow erase what you have been through. Perhaps it's perceived as an energetic recompense from a system that is supposed to protect you. Perhaps it is a way to keep you quiet since money can be seen as a sign of power; when you sue and win, you have reached a victory. However, there can be many reasons why you have chosen not to go the route of suing. While we know holding faulty practitioners accountable for wrongdoings is important, and can be done simply by writing a review or filing a complaint with the hospital where you gave birth, I want you to release any shame you might be harboring. If not suing was your choice, it may be because you are highly aware of the following reasons why suing was not going to bring you peace or change the trajectory to healing.

Reliving the memory

You may have decided not to sue because repeating the experience in front of a jury with the process of potentially not being believed is something you wouldn't be able to live with. Repeating over and over the details of a horrid experience isn't good for your nervous system and can make it difficult for you to move forward.

Confronting your practitioner

In a system and society where it is ingrained that our practitioners are more qualified to make certain decisions regarding our health, it can seem intimidating and maybe even audacious to want to confront your practitioner. Maybe you are not interested in engaging in any more power struggles.

Fear of Betraying the Group

When we talk about the maternal mortality rate of the United States, we can automatically go into the tropes of racism and how the medical industrial complex is killing Black women. However, what my experience highlighted was how threatening it can be to experience a preventable surgery at the hands of someone who comes from your race, particularly if it is considered a minority group. It is quite understandable that you would harbor some fear around bringing attention to a false move made by this practitioner. It is no secret that racism is alive and well within the medical system, here in this country. However, affirming that poor care is not always about race, but always about the structure of medical care, is not for the fainthearted. Having just emerged from the experience, don't feel ashamed should you choose to focus all your energies towards healing. Should you submit reviews to your hospital or birthing center as a result of what has happened to you? Absolutely, if you feel the courage to do so.

Hiring an Attorney

When friends, family members, or even strangers randomly suggest you should have just gone and pursued legal action, they might just be oblivious to what the cost is to seek legal action. Hiring legal counsel designated to handle the proceedings of suing a hospital or medical group totally depends upon the fees they charge for litigation and whether or not they will represent a client through something called contingency fees. There are also state laws in place that can impact an attorney's ability to accept a contingency based case.

Feeling Silenced by Money

If you have emerged from surgery and decided that your experience deserves to be shared with others to help them, much like my experience has found its way onto paper and into this book, perhaps you feel taking legal action and actually winning would push you into silence. There is this unexplored after-effect of what is socially expected from you when you win a case. You should take your money and keep it moving. Keeping quiet might not be what you were after to begin with. Learning how to express yourself, reclaim your voice from being violated is your goal and the primary reason why you are reading this book.

Money Doesn't Heal the Core Wound

Yes money does pay bills, and provides assistance for the daily needs we need met that injuries interfere with. However, I strongly believe it does not heal a core wound of trust being violated nor does receiving money for an offense provide root chakra safety. Receiving a lump sum of money may seem like the proper jurisdictional response. However, spiritually it may not grant answers around "why" and "what's next."

Regardless of which of these reasons have been your own, please allow yourself to be comforted by the fact that it is absolutely none of anyone's business why you did not feel compelled to pursue legal action. Refusing to pursue legal action as a means to ease the burden of the trauma caused does not and cannot cancel out your right to heal, and become whole.

Whatever reason you have chosen is valid. And sharing your story, once you have gone through the entire process of reassembling a whole and healed version of yourself, is indeed the greatest form of retribution you could ever seek to achieve. So sis, if you find yourself loathing and drowning in regret, shame, and fear, remember you are only poisoning your precious body. Let those narratives go. Do not allow yourself to shrink in embarrassment the way I did during that baseless conversation. Extend whatever forgiveness you can muster to those around you who have no understanding or idea what you have been through. Do not waste any energy on trying to convince them or defend yourself. The only thing you are responsible for is investing that necessary chi into becoming the most restored version of yourself, and the best version of a mother your child could ever have.

Part II.

—

Steering Your Path to Healing

Chapter 4

Understanding the World of Complementary & Alternative Healing

———

"I wasn't raised like that Laura. I think you have more exposure to the "natural" way of doing things," Marie said, shrugging her shoulders as she dipped a piece of fried calamari in the tangy tartar sauce we were sharing as we waited for our burgers to arrive. Marie and I decided to make a quick trip to one of our favorite burger spots for a much needed "mommy moment" when she began sharing the details of a recent meltdown she'd had around trying to navigate a scheduling dilemma for her two daughters. Listening intently, but noticing the overwhelming emotion present in her body language, I made a suggestion preceded by a question. "Have you considered trying another modality of healing to see if you can release these emotions on a deeper level?" I suggested she see a Reiki practitioner who could target things on a much more somatic level. I just got the sense, this not having been the first time discussing emotional upsets stemming from the birth she'd had, that perhaps a more energetic approach could be deeply supportive. However, as is so common in certain circles, stepping outside of what conventional medicine considers traditional forms of care is such a taboo topic. It is often assumed that to take a route not celebrated by mainstream media is to be playing Russian roulette with your health. It is considered borderline neglectful if you try a path and instead of getting better right away, a healing crisis occurs first where you might experience more of a system upset or purging before completely feeling better.

Knowing this, I wasn't at all offended by her response because going to counseling or seeing a talk therapist was an amazing first step in working on healing the emotional issues around her birth. One study revealed that in a cohort of 29,601 women, only 9% of white, new mothers sought mental health therapy as a means of support postpartum. These percentages are even smaller in communities of color with reportedly 4% Black/African American mothers, and 5% Latinx mothers sought therapy. As a Black woman, I don't at all find these numbers to be startling considering how in chapter two we discussed the way Black women were historically treated when giving birth. Seeking therapy for postnatal post traumatic stress was non-existent and the response of simply praying your way through the pain is an inherently generational and community-oriented solution. There is also the fear of being labeled as unfit to mother, possibly having the system misconstrue your feelings of sadness or righteous anger for early signs of a clinical mental health disorder. It is widely known amongst Black and other women of color communities just how dangerous it can be to self and family to try and establish autonomy. Trying to reject a diagnosis that requires a mother to take medication can sometimes be seen by a medical professional as failing to act in compliance. Therefore, to take a step towards going to therapy to engage in Briefs Solution Focused or Person-Centered techniques is certainly one thing, but to go a step further to seek support from a non-traditional, more frequency based manner such as Biofeedback, could definitely cause a stir. I knew this was the undercurrent to Marie's response at dinner and many other mothers who reflect her desire to get better but feel uncertain about trying a different or complementary path. But if your story resembles that of Sarah's where the fear of flatlining during a c-section like your mother did is generational, trying a more body-work, somatic, energy-based modality would prove to be quite beneficial because these serve to shift the trauma from the auric field in a way that is limited in more talk-based, conventional approaches.

You might be at a place on your postpartum journey where you're investigating what path to restoration resonates best. Perhaps your family has a history of drug abuse or chemical solutions that have wreaked havoc on your body in the past, or perhaps you simply want to feel better using a non-chemical approach to healing. When it comes to what is considered non-traditional, holistic, or alternative approaches, much of your decision-making might get colored by how your family of origin or your newly created family feels about them—not necessarily objective information. You might also be overwhelmed by what some in social media spaces have dubbed the Wellness Industrial Complex, which prides itself on doing tons of showing, but not necessarily enough telling when it comes to how to actually solve health issues and discomforts. That is to say, not everyone is properly practicing within their scope of practice, which only stokes the fires of fear that much more. Wanting to try a more holistic, preventative approach without enough knowledge or proper information can lead to shaming, being made to feel intimidated, or even ridiculed for choosing a particular path. Your mind might swirl with questions like, "Well, should I try Reiki? Yoga therapy? Should I go to traditional talk therapy? Do I actually need meds? Is it more prayer I am in need of? How do I know? Will oils truly help me? Is it a change of diet? Is it my environment?" The thing to consider first is that every mother comes to healing at different stages of the postpartum journey, next is understanding that we each have an individual and unique constitution that governs how well each of us responds to different types of therapy. While this perspective isn't always explored in conventional approaches and there can be a heavy lean towards the inclusion of medication for managing symptoms of postnatal post traumatic stress, being considerate of each person's constitution is a foundation for choosing a holistic approach. This perspective is also why I have modeled the different aspects of the method in a way where there is room for you to explore what will work most efficiently depending on where you personally stand on your current path. With that being said, where you are and what's showing up for you should be taken into consideration before anyone else's opinion. For instance, when I first gave birth, telemedicine was not as popular as it is today. Therefore, going to see a therapist would require me to travel physically. In the dead of winter, with fresh stitches and while taking care of my two children, heading out proved to be impossible and an approach I simply didn't want. Talking about what happened wasn't the problem, dealing with all the unexpected changes and halts were.

What is most important before deciding on a particular path to restoration for your postpartum journey is to understand how each approach can support you in healing from c-section birth trauma and how each addresses things very differently. Choosing Reiki over talk therapy or hours of prayer at your pastor's doesn't make you less of a believer or negligent. Having education on different forms of healing techniques allows the faith you have in your Creator to manifest healing in your body and subsequently, your life. You are not defiant for being honest about your limitations, be it physically, financially, or whatever else—the goal is to feel grounded in the ways you do choose to activate your healing. With a lack of information or perhaps awareness, we've unfortunately been indoctrinated into believing someone else should always have more authority over our mothering bodies, implying that "if we don't do this, then this will happen." And when these types of very subliminally frightening phrases are used, you can be sure fear mongering is taking place, rather than a desire for you to be truly well. While we know conventional medicine has done so much for humanity in terms of peer-reviewed research and advancements, there is still room for the application of ancient traditions that err on the side of being non-invasive—modalities you should have the knowledge to discern about. And in this vein, you can make whole, informed decisions around what will best serve you, what can be merged together, or what simply will not work for you.

I often cringe when I share the healing properties of herbs, oils, or crystals for support and am met with scrunched up noses, and the immediate correlation of these approaches with witchcraft or a lack of scientific weight to be deemed applicable for promoting one's health and wellness. However, peer-reviewed medical research has begun to confirm what traditional healers, naturopaths, and shamans of old have known since the beginning of time- and that is the properties of nature, including herbs, essential oils, and flower essences contain properties designed to support the body's innate ability to heal given the appropriate circumstances and environment. Using herbs and essential oils are a non-synthetic way of providing the body with the additional support it needs when fighting things like stress and grief.

Gemstone therapy, sometimes referred to as "Crystal Healing," while not supported by clinical, peer-reviewed literature due to an insufficient comprehensive understanding on disease states, is recognized as a complementary medicine approach to promoting a shift in mood that in some regions is preferred to prescription medication. Perhaps this is due to the vibrational properties of different gemstones and their impact on your subtle body energy, what I referred to earlier as your auric field, as the body is made up of electromagnetic energy. Scripturally, there is mention of the use of gemstones in the book of Exodus. Precious stones such as carnelian, beryl, turquoise, lapis lazuli, and others are mentioned, and were used as part of priestly garments further demonstrating their significance on promoting wellness of the psychological, subtle body energy type. It is scriptural that you are not to worship or practice any form of idolatry, meaning we all acknowledge the Source of all healing, but it does not condemn use of the Earth's properties to promote health and wellness. It is also important that we acknowledge that everything on this earthly plane has both shadow and light. The intention behind what you engage in is the driving factor for what aspect you activate.

In the example of counseling therapy or even psychiatric care, we can see the shadow revealed when practitioners engage in power struggles with patients and their families, suggesting they know what's best, or when factors of racism or discrimination surface through treatment options. We should also be aware of how prescription medication recommended through treatment protocols come with tons of side effects that most patients accept as part of the managing of their symptoms. This can be an extremely triggering decision for a mother who in the past may have experienced tons of hormonal struggles after deciding to come off of birth control, only to learn the most recommended way to heal from postnatal post traumatic stress is to get back on pharmaceuticals. Just this year, the American Psychological Association released a public statement in the form of an apology for racist practices being at the root of their research practices and methods. Historically, here in the States, theories around health, genetics, and even the realm of mental illness were derived from very racist, eugenics-led ideas, making it incredibly difficult for Black women, and other women of color to seek treatment. While I would never suggest every mental health counselor or psychotherapist has a practice based on racist principles, as this form of therapy is all about the desire to help others rewrite their personal stories through the application of theories in a supported way, I will say this revelation makes it all the more important for you to avoid making uninformed decisions driven predominantly by fear. Fear of what your family will say, fear of what your friends might say, fear in general.

When it comes to talk therapy or what is formally known as mental health counseling and psychotherapy, it is also not a one-size-fits-all type of experience. Therapists use a range of techniques or theoretical approaches in their goal to help clients cope through major transitions, gain insight, and gain emotional awareness to change attitude and behaviors. Each technique is rooted in theory centered around the belief that the client is competent and has the cure to her problems, but needs empathy, trust, and the safe space to retrieve it. Sessions focus around using one or more approaches to help clients talk their way through suffering and into a healthier, more fulfilled life. For example, CBT or Cognitive Behavioral Therapy is an approach that helps clients identify core beliefs and assumptions around their experiences while providing interventions designed to help them unlearn maladaptive behaviors, replacing them with adaptive behaviors. By helping you change the way you think about something, the goal is to help you behave differently about it as well. An example of this would be in stress management and developing strategies to cope.

One of my favorite techniques to incorporate when working with mothers stems from a Positive Psychology model I used during my time as a school counselor. It is called The Indivisible Self Positive Psychology model. Created by psychologists Thomas Sweeney and Jane E. Meyers, "The Indivisible Self" is a particular approach to mental wellness that takes into account all the factors, personal and societal, that can affect a person's path to healing emotionally. It is one

[5] American Psychological Association. (2021). Apology to people of color for APA's role in promoting, perpetuating, and failing to challenge racism, racial discrimination, and human hierarchy in U. S. https://www.apa.org/about/policy/racism-apology

of the models that inspired me to really think about how often we as mothers struggle to heal. This is because many practitioners, bound by their scope of practice, can only work to help mothers cope, but not necessarily heal, because the trauma isn't just on a purely psychological level. When overall coping cannot happen because the amount of change and disruption ahead for the mother causes her to feel stuck or blatantly incapable of making progress, psychotherapists may feel medication is the next best step. But many forget that most of the load falls on us: our families depend on us, and yet we still have little to no control over things like paid leave or when daycare costs skyrocket to the point where you or your spouse is forced to quit work to care for the beautiful family you've just begun creating. Our world, particularly as millennials, looks quite different than that of our parents. We can all heartily agree the days of having your neighbor from down the block or across the way "watch your kids for a few hours" are far and few between. This is why it can be so hard for some to move beyond the storylines explored through traditional talk therapy. This is why a mother like Marie, who believed her emergency c-section was all her fault, might have a great mental health counselor or therapist, but struggle to experience complete healing. In today's society, care for the physical and spiritual bodies are just as important, if not as vital as the mental/emotional body. They simply cannot be separated as they have been in the past. As a stressed, but widely-respected art dealer, Marie could have benefited from the rebalancing of sacral chakra energy and what it represents– addressing the fear of losing creative and fiscal control of her life.

Daily maintenance of our health and wellness is one thing, but when your life is turned inside out from the impact of something as unexpected as birth trauma, specifically c-section birth trauma, healing must take place multidimensionally. But don't feel guilty if this knowledge isn't innate. You also shouldn't feel guilty if you aren't sure where to start, especially when there is a ton of information swirling around from just about every corner of the internet stratosphere. Becoming proactive in choosing a method and modality you feel aligned with becomes overwhelming. I want you to feel empowered so I am going to break down some of the most popular and beneficial forms of therapy, from the best understood—conventional talk therapy— to what has been considered alternative and might seem a little foreign. Listed below, you'll find several bodywork and energy medicine modalities that have been proven by scientific research to support the alleviation of root causes linked to great emotional imbalances. These approaches are naturopathic in nature, meaning they support the body's innate ability to heal itself given the right conditions and they target different systems of the body that have direct influence over the state of emotional health and wellbeing. I'll have further resources listed in the index for further exploration.

Ready? Let's go.

Counseling

An umbrella covering many fields—such as social work, school counseling (from which my training stems), psychology, mental health and clinical counseling, pastoral counseling, and briefly, psychiatry—counseling supports clients in an intensive and personal process. The main focus with this form of therapy is to help you cope with normal problems, even if the problems that seem normal are much more complex in nature. When you enter a counselor-client relationship, your counselor's goal is to build positive rapport, use listening skills to understand your story, and obtain a common goal to achieve, one that usually involves rewriting aspects of your story. A quality or experienced counselor will work with you through moments of resistance, supporting you via the use of myriad theory-based approaches geared towards helping the client resolve issues of the mind that can impact how you feel and/or perceive your reality. Sessions can last up to an hour and client-counselor relationships can span years depending on the nature of the client's needs and the counselor's theoretical approach and style.

Reiki

A non-invasive, energy-healing technique which originated in Japan, Reiki involves a practitioner setting pure and positive intention for healing and being used as a channel for Source energy. Literally meaning Rei "Light," and Ki "Source"), this modality is similar to the Christian concept of "laying hands." However, you do not need to be of any specific belief system to be a recipient of this type of session. Just as with any other type of therapy, picking a practitioner should begin with your gut feeling around compatibility. A session of Reiki involves a trained Reiki Master laying the client on a practicing table. The client is always fully clothed during sessions and is typically asked beforehand what some key discomforts have been prior to the session. Using certain hand positions, the practitioner will work with the client's auric field to allow the universal life force energy to begin healing. This can include either focusing on a specific location on the body or working on the entire energy field. This form of therapy can bring deep relaxation to the body as it is cleared of debris, negative emotion, shock, and even trauma, which, when left unaddressed, can manifest as physical symptoms. For a mother working through the different elements of c-section birth trauma, this is a gentle and non-invasive way of bringing healing to the mind, body, and spirit. Sessions tend to last anywhere from 45 minutes to an hour. To find a practitioner and to learn more about their training, please reference the resource guide at the back of the book.

Sound Healing

Music lifts. Music transcends. Ever wonder why? Well, music is composed of notes and these notes carry a certain frequency or vibration that, when heard, can create various effects on the body. At a certain frequency, the effects on the body are positive because they induce the feelings of hope, love, peace, calm and other positive thoughts. Sound Healing is a form of energy healing because it involves the practitioner using certain frequencies to bring balance to the energy field and eventually your physical body. This is why when you go into certain environments, such as a spa, the music playing is usually classical or instrumental, and tends to invoke serenity. This is intentional and that is what this type of therapy provides. Through the use of special bowls and tuning forks, the practitioner strikes notes to clear the energy field and to invoke feelings of calmness. This can ultimately support the prevention of stress, allowing you to remain in a parasympathetic state and allowing your immune system to reboot. Your feelings and thoughts, related to your organs, are a powerful driver behind your ability to cultivate wellness, as stress from the birth and stress around moving forward with postpartum life can adversely affect and even weaken the immune system's functioning. Emotions lodged in your auric field and cellular vibration can get a chance to shift through this healing modality.

Reflexology

A Naturopathic modality, Reflexology is both a science and form of therapy derived from the concept that our feet have reflex points directly corresponding to all the organs and parts of the body. Through the appropriate stimulation of these reflexes, blockages to the organs caused by a lack of fresh blood flow are released. The release of this discord leads to improved health and wellness. Developed by physiotherapist Eunice D. Ingham, the practice of reflexology is one that allows the practitioner to connect directly with the health of your organs based on the soreness or tenderness of a particular reflex point when pressure is applied. When it comes to c-section birth trauma healing, this therapy can be beneficial on many levels. From supporting the organs involved in the surgery as they heal, to releasing tension emotionally, this therapy involves the practitioner working along the points or ten zones of the body for approximately 2-3 minutes each.

Acupuncture

A healing technique of Traditional Chinese Medicine, acupuncture works on the premise that wellness is created and supported by correcting the flow of "qi" or vital force eenergy throughout the body. Acupuncture is used by practitioners to stimulate the circulation of this vital force energy through 14 major pathways, which are called meridians, throughout the body. When the flow of energy along these channels is blocked or sluggish, the corresponding organs are adversely impacted, including how you experience a variety of emotions connected to each organ. This is because proper blood flow nourishes your organs. Through the insertion of hair-thin needles at what are called "chi gateways," practitioners stimulate this flow. While the insertion of the needles is said to be painless, some soreness or numbness may be present depending upon the condition of the meridian and its corresponding acupoint. A session involves the practitioner making observations of your general presentation and your tongue, taking your pulse, and asking you questions around lifestyle and daily habits. This is a wonderful therapy choice for supporting the rebalancing of the entire system from c-section birth trauma, as it helps to expel deeper emotions lodged in the different organs. This healing technique also activates your parasympathetic nervous system, bringing calm to the emotional body. The ultimate goal of this form of therapy is to bring balance back to the entire system, which again stimulates healthy immune functioning, and allows nature to steer her course of bringing healing to the mind, body, and spirit.

Aromatherapy

Also considered a Naturopathic modality here in the West, aromatherapy is an ancient healing therapy that involves using the aromatic qualities of plants, in the form of essential oils, to elicit responses from the limbic system of the brain, directly impacting mood and memory. The limbic system also influences hormone production, the immune system, and the nervous system. The chemical molecules of each essential oil interact differently with this part of the brain, supporting different bodily functions related to these systems. This happens primarily through the inhalation of an oil and its molecules travel up the nasal pathways and make contact with the olfactory bulb; the beginning of the limbic system. Topical application, where you dilute drops of an oil with a carrier oil, is another therapeutic approach. Topically, the oil's molecules penetrate the skin and enter the bloodstream supporting your internal organs and the lymphatic system. These molecules also travel to the lungs, enter the bloodstream, and positively act on your individual cells! Some essential oils have antiseptic and antibacterial qualities such as Melaleuca, while others are used during massage to promote circulation. Essential oils and their scents are generally grouped into different categories based on their properties and part of the plant. For example, citrus oils such as Lime, Bergamot, and Wild Orange are used to stimulate positivity, happiness, and self-esteem. This is because these oils' chemical components stimulate the release of neurotransmitters. Essential oils such as Lavender, Roman Chamomile, and Rose are used for more calming, soothing, and relaxing qualities, whereas more wooded scents like Cedarwood and Vetiver are used for their grounding qualities. Inhalation or diffusion through a diffuser are generally the most efficient manners when it comes to mood management, while topical is best used for other types of ailments such as burns, circulation problems, and much more. In chapter seven, I share how using essential oils can support activating the parasympathetic state for continued calm.

Massage

While this form of therapy automatically screams physical relaxation, massage therapy also provides relief from emotional tension and so much more. This type of therapy improves circulation, supports the healing of soft tissue after injury and helps to control pain, which can bring immense emotional comfort to the body. A session of massage involves laying undressed, but covered by designated blankets, on a warmed massage table, and the parts of the body being massaged are the only parts left uncovered. The room is usually dimly lit to create a relaxing atmosphere. Instrumental or classical music might be playing and you might be offered a cup of room temperature water with lemon prior to your session starting. This helps to support the body in releasing toxins pre-massage. There are different types of massage including Swedish, deep-tissue, and hot-stone, which target specific needs, and you are able to speak with your massage therapist about concerns you have, including any areas that are particularly sensitive.

---

[6] Stengler, Mark, et al. "Aromatherapy Basics." Prescription for Natural Cures: A Self-Care Guide for Treating Health Problems with Natural Remedies Including Diet, Nutrition, Supplements, and Other Holistic Methods, Turner Publishing Company, Nashville, TN, 2016, pp. 773–773.

Craniosacral Therapy

A very gentle and noninvasive therapy form, Craniosacral therapy, is based on the concept that the circulation of craniosacral fluid, which surrounds and supports the brain and spinal cord, has a specific rhythm. This rhythm is created from the continuous draining and refilling of the fluid. This rhythm can get disrupted by events such as trauma, after which neurotransmitters are unable to correctly communicate with the brain. First developed by osteopath William Sutherland, this therapy involves the manipulation of the bones of the skull and spine. This manipulation releases tension that impairs this natural rhythmic oscillation and brings it back into balance. This type of session involves the practitioner instructing the client to lay flat on their back while gently pressing certain fascial points on the back of the head, neck, and sometimes waist. Gently touching these points, the practitioner waits to feel the rhythm of the fluid's expansion and contraction, and wherever it is out of balance, their trained touch, resets it. This process brings the entire body back to what is called a still point, greatly providing relief from birth trauma effects such as TMJ, headaches, and even anxiety.

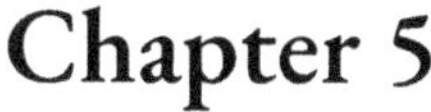

Chapter 5

The Throat Chakra & Call To Surrender

I want you to think back to that time you were in say the third or fourth grade, and something unpleasant happened to you while in school. It could be a lunch lady making a snide comment about the way your mom made your lunch; it could be that you worked super hard on a project only to have an adult undermine your efforts because he or she believed someone did better than you. How did these types of experiences make you feel, if you can recall? Were you given permission to talk about it or did you feel it more appropriate to keep it quiet? Keep yourself from having to speak up against a "Goliath" of sorts? Did you feel like it would be too tedious to get your parents involved?

So many questions, I know, but chances are, if you think long enough about these questions, you might be able to remember just when your throat chakra energy was being developed. And through these experiences, you unconsciously began learning how to operate in your personal voice, and here, we might be able to pinpoint the first time you had your throat chakra energy challenged. This is because here is where you learned to communicate what was in your heart and saw how the outside world would respond to your truth. Here is where you began learning how to operate in your personal will by communicating what you desired to happen in the world around you. Here is where you learned the power of your personal voice and what the cost of speaking with integrity might be.

The throat chakra, located at the throat region of the body, is linked to your larynx, vocal cords, ears, and mouth. The throat chakra is also connected to the thyroid and parathyroids which have an important relationship to hormonal control throughout the body. Your thyroid regulates metabolism which impacts weight loss and gain, heat production in your body (cold hands, cold feet), energy in the body, and most importantly, the production of calcitonin which regulates calcium levels in the bloodstream. Without a proper balance of calcium in your body, healthy bones, tissues, and blood clotting is impossible. The throat chakra is one of seven bodies of energy that spin. These bodies of energy move upward along the body and vibrate in a way that collects (or sends) information through the skin. This is why what you hear or allow yourself to hear (words, sounds, music, information) determines how and with what words you choose to respond to the world around you.

You might not realize it, but you have energy inside of you moving faster than the speed of light, transmitting information to these spinning wheels. These wheels influence your mind, body, and spirit, depending on what is being exchanged in and around you. You also have something called an auric field surrounding your physical body, which connects the chakras. These aspects—mind, body, and spirit—are interconnected, and chakras reflect the vibrational battery connecting all three and act as a connector to the endocrine system. The endocrine system sends its signals depending on how you are responding to external stressors and circumstances. So for instance, when you have a relationship with your practitioner that becomes filled with violation—she wants to perform an exam on your womb that you aren't comfortable with, but for compliance's sake you allow it—the stress from suppressing your true feelings in this interaction can impact the hormonal communication between your thyroid, pituitary and adrenal glands. Your throat chakra begins the journey of doing things for survival, outward mobility, and negotiating matters of the heart. Here, we navigate the balance between what we fear will happen if we choose Divine guidance, what will happen when we make choices out of fear, and what happens if our ability to choose is thwarted altogether. An example of this is how we as mothers are constantly faced with the challenge of practicing self-advocacy regarding the needs of our families and what we intuitively know to be the right path against a system that constantly challenges our integrity and internal wisdom.

In those particular moments and through those types of experiences where the fear of systemically enforced consequences seem overwhelming or sifting through the confusion that a violation of our choices brings, we learn what it means to "not rock the boat." And by that, I mean we learn how to keep authority figures from getting in trouble, or worse, keep ourselves from getting in trouble by challenging them in front of others. In this respect, the throat chakra is all about the power of communication and how we can lose that power, sometimes without it even being our own fault. Here in this chakra, we begin to deal with the internalizing of these experiences and the seeds of guilt and shame planted for not speaking up enough in the midst of confrontations or events when our personal authority is unjustly challenged. It is at this energetic point of the body, different from the more physical ones that precede it, that our thought life becomes more disrupted; the domino effect of behaving in a way that demonstrates having our entire energy system disrupted without even knowing it. We just become more talkative competitive, more loud and brash, talkative, more vindictive and punishing, more doubtful and self-sabotaging.

This is what happened to Nathalie, who at a very young age competed in an athletic competition. Although she had rigorously trained, and fairly beat her competition, an adult flat out told her that another athlete deserved to win the trophy over her. Both devastated and humiliated by the reprimand, she didn't challenge this adult or the absurdity of her comments. No, instead, this young girl grew into a woman who constantly second guessed her accomplishments or pushed herself to the edge of preparation for fear that someone would come out of the bushes and ambush her. While this experience and many others like it do subtle damage on external things like self-esteem, they also impact the entire energy system. Because everything in our bodies is connected, the learned and internalized lesson to keep quiet continues to throw other interrelated chakras out of balance because the shame we begin to feel doesn't get resolved. Instead, the imbalance begins to drive other aspects of our behavior.

This is why so many women tend to shy away from discussion around how a negative birthing experience, especially one rooted in power struggle, so deeply impacts them. This is why it can seem so easy to initially brush off the experience and replace shock with gratitude as we discussed in chapter one. Much like not challenging the authority figure who violates, leaning towards infinite gratitude to God or the Divine feels more acceptable than calling out an offense for what it is, a violation.

This is why so many women develop issues around their thyroid and parathyroid glands, affecting weight gain and loss, and even calcium levels related to bone and structural health. We often write these off as simply pre-menopausal or menopausal issues, but the way we manage our birthing history deeply impacts this area of our lives. Issues around immune system dysfunction can be linked to the development of conditions like fibromyalgia, rheumatoid arthritis, and gout. Issues can arise in the throat, thyroid, esophagus, teeth, gums, ears, voice (pitch/volume), neck, and finally, the tonsils. This is caused not only by the quality of what we're saying, but what we aren't saying and why. Proper functioning of personal expression via the throat chakra can come down to the answers to the following questions:

- **Who am I offending by sharing this truth?**
- **Who will stop loving me as a result of sharing this?**
- **Who will get in trouble as a result of my speaking up and out?**
- **Who am I betraying by sharing my story? By advocating on the behalf of those whom I share this experience with?**
- **Who is going to judge or reject me for sharing an experience shared by the collective, but has given me a different outcome?**

This is all because, through these early experiences, we receive the message that it is not safe to communicate. Memories locked in the limbic system can tend to replay themselves anytime we think about challenging those in authority. We question whether the hassle and, subsequently, the embarrassment, will be worth it. While a medical practitioner in the form of an obstetrician doesn't have authority over you, once under their care, it can be very difficult to feel or experience otherwise. From the start of the relationship it is usually made very clear that you are the patient and don't always have the permission to vocalize an opinion or preference contrary to theirs. When we internalize the message that it is unsafe to communicate our personal truth, not only does a cascade of other issues surface, but our ability to trust our Creator through divine redirection becomes obstructed. We can become stuck in our thinking around how to move forward, a quality of a depleted spleen meridian which we discussed earlier. Confusion and even feelings of abandonment may cause us to feel unsure about how we can heal from this experience, how to find meaning, or even further, how this process could ever serve a greater purpose in our lives.

However, as we begin to reflect on our relationship to Divine prior to the birth, we can gently unpack these questions:

- **How am I healing my matrilineal lineage by speaking my truth?**

- **Is there anyone else in my lineage who suffered from being made to feel like keeping quiet to keep the peace?**

- **Did someone in my lineage pay a heavy price, i.e. face death, excommunication, imprisonment, alienation, or community isolation for speaking on something taboo?**

As we look at it from a spiritual lens and consider what type of testimony might be possible from this experience, we begin the necessary inner work of creating a new narrative about ourselves—one that is free from shame, guilt, anger, remorse, and self-condemnation.

With this focus on inner work, forgiveness of self, and physical healing, we can still be advocates for others, but from a place where we have nothing to prove, no one to impress, and even better, no need to seek to live in an identity of woundedness. Here in this place of surrender, we lay down the extreme spectrums of keeping too quiet or lashing out. Here, we can settle in to unpack.

When I think about what it means to be put back together after experiencing c-section birth trauma, it is obvious that we are not coming from a place that is unharmed. The experience in and of itself is harmful. However, experiencing wholeness as a mother means gathering all the fragmented pieces of ourselves and our experience, sitting with each piece and working through as if reconstructing the glass window panes of a church. We need to sit with the sharp edges that could very well cut us and, using noninvasive tools to buffer, reshape, and soften those pieces, reconnect with a much more beautiful, robust, and deeply opened version of ourselves. As I am writing this, I cannot help but smile as I reflect on the various sharp edges that needed buffing before I could even think to have this conversation. These are the sharp edges that threatened to keep my voice quiet, shy, embarrassed, and ashamed around the experience of this birth and its life-altering impact. But they would eventually become polished, even redefined, once I began to make room for a nervous system that needed slowing down and care. This led me to identify the first part of the method as Rest.

Then, adopting a new relationship with my physical self beyond losing weight or snapping back, I would slowly explore different foods as they related to the systems of my body in need of repair most, primarily the digestive, nervous, and endocrine systems, which would serve as the foundation to an overall more balanced me. Along with external, beauty-related changes I would experience around my hair and teeth specifically, I would also learn how to cultivate my sexuality and sensuality in this period. This is what led me to call the next portion of the method, Replenish.

Finally, in my focus on inner work and acceptance around the major shifts created by this birthing experience, I surrendered to time, and used the Coping Self aspect of the Indivisible Self Model- the positive psychology theory mentioned earlier, and deep reflection, along with prayer and chakra work, to unzip all the areas of my life. Careful reconstruction would help me to determine to use my voice for healing and advocacy, rather than rage and revenge. This portion of the method is called Reevaluate.

Part III.

———

The Whole Mother Method

Chapter 6

REST

———

It's no secret our culture has become obsessed with throwing around the word "rest" as a catch phrase of some sort. But if you too happen to be a millennial generation mother, you know this now-commercialized attempt to get us to pay attention to something other than "grinding" isn't something that is out of context. As members of what has been defined by researchers and economists alike as "knowledge economy," millennial generation mothers are part of a society that capitalizes and literally functions off the productivity of what we know—and even "fun" things or "restful" activities have been turned into things to know, and ways to make money.

Since the 1980's, American society has shifted from an industrial approach—think assembly lines and factories—to a more technology-based approach. This explosion and expansion—think computers, the internet, and life as we know it—has also caused the need for higher education to secure positions that can compete in global markets. According to a 2012 U.S. Chamber of Commerce General Foundation research study on millennials, 68% of high school graduates were enrolled at a four-year university, 58% were expected to receive a Bachelor's degree, while 27 % sought to enroll in a graduate degree program. As a generation, we are noted to be the most educated in history, but also the most fiscally in debt from student loans. This constant need to learn, share, and compete in order to live, combined with the pressure of an already unstable economy, debilitating student loan debt, skyrocketing rent, and an ambiguous retirement plan, has created an environment where social media accounts everywhere are begging you to lean in to whatever restorative practices you can get your hands on, while the very culture resists it.

This backdrop for generational burnout is eloquently documented in The Burnout Generation, by Anne Helen Petersen, in which Peterson breaks down how exhausting life has become for many mothers of my time. Scrolling through apps like what is formerly known as Twitter, keeps many moms feeling bad about the world because while there's an instinctual desire to use productivity to help create long-term solutions to societal issues that abound, she cannot help but notice how what's seen as the productive thing to do comes at the cost of neglecting the importance of filling her own maternal cup. Surrendering to this importance can often read to the greater productive world around her that motherhood has now absorbed her. Petersen highlights just how much we've been taught to value our ability to navigate unending to-do lists and action-oriented planning that would hopefully yield us capable of not missing a beat. But what caught my attention about the research was the lack of research around how millennial generation mothers are supposed to navigate the ever changing waters of the postpartum journey while still being members of the all-consuming fire that is knowledge economy. It's no wonder mothers are screaming from an exhaustion that a nap cannot cure. We need such a more substantial kind of rest.

As a mother recovering from the post traumatic stress from my c-section, trying to contextualize rest meant tackling some of our culture's worst, most deeply ingrained teachings around worth and productivity. And still today, in 2022, your need for rest in the stage of your postpartum journey post-surgery might look very different from what mine looked like back in 2016. The fact of the matter is that making rest about unpacking the things that were sending my nervous system into overdrive was going to be key to getting to a place of mind-body-spirit wellness.

For me, contextualizing rest came in the form of needing to once again learn how to slow down without feeling like I was falling behind. Rest needed to address some deep-seated fears around loss, around being unable to be the productive adult I enjoyed being prior to this life-altering surgery and experience. Rest, for me, meant learning how to use techniques that could strengthen, soothe, and ground my very empathic and highly sensitive nature while allowing me to navigate some of the deepest aspects of the emotions we tend to shadowban in our society. Rest meant I needed help to get back in my body when I started feeling uncertain, ungrounded, and even cornered about the details of my once very well-planned, organized future. From where I was standing, everything that I had planned was slipping through my fingers like sand.

Case in point: on one morning in December of 2017, I woke up to my toddler stirring, giving me the routine signal he'd be waking shortly and would begin his squeal of urgency around needing breakfast almost immediately. Gently removing his brother's sleepy grip of my nipple, rounding out the first of what would become a three-year breastfeeding journey, I tucked him back into his bed. My heart beating at a rapid-fire pace, and I quietly slipped off the bed and into my slippers as quickly as I could— a daily practice I had learned to apply if I wanted the day to start unscathed. As I gently shut the bedroom door, I began praying silently, begging God to keep me from crying for the day. It had been two months since we moved into a totally new neighborhood somewhat abruptly, after living very closely with my parents, and I was feeling exhausted.

We had settled into a somewhat gentrified area of a suburb I was already familiar with, but I had no idea how childless this particular neighborhood really was or how isolated it would make me feel. The daily nervousness I carried from being in an area where there was so little presence of other parents of small children had begun to wear on me. Another thing that began to wear on my nervous system was the new identity of being a stay-at-home mom. I had never taken a class or watched a movie on what it would be like to be a stay-at-home-mom in the suburbs of New York City. Let me remind you this was in 2017, way before the time of pandemic, when it was automatically assumed that a mom as young as I was would be working during the day and my children in daycare. Some of the nonverbal, often subtle expressions of the people in the area reminded me of this daily.

Wanting to adjust to this season and environment, I tried taking both boys to the local playground. While it might seem like I'm reaching with what I'm about to share, I kid you not, it didn't matter whether I showed up to the nearby playground in dress casual or University alumni para, I would get asked regularly if I was my boys' nanny. Apparently, it was unfathomable for me to be a stay-at-home mom. Due to my prior experience of immediately returning to work after my first pregnancy, this was brand new territory. Feeling overwhelmed by constantly having to start my sentences with replies like, "Well I was actually a full-time school counselor, but my near-death c-section forced me to take more time off than expected," or "No, these are my boys and I'm in the middle of finishing my first manuscript," the trips proved to be less therapeutic than I'd hoped for. Actually, either response left me feeling somewhat ashamed in the moment. It felt like my body had failed me since I hadn't healed in the record 12 weeks we are always promised. That, and everyone I knew was busy working or simply being productive outside the home.

In these awkward paused moments, I would be met with stares of sympathy or overall confusion. While I would usually get awkwardly uncomfortable with a complete stranger's sympathy, telling them "no, it's okay, I'm fine," it was usually the confusion I could resonate with or better understand. It was just not a common thing to hear a woman living in New York, was taking off "more time" from work to heal from a near-death c-section. I say this because with maternal health and mortality now being a major topic of national concern, I know I am not the only woman who's had to recover from a traumatic c-section. I also know with the lack of policy supporting maternity leave, taking a "longer break" could cost you your job, much like it cost me mine.

To keep from having to engage in these often draining and limitation-reminding conversations, I gradually stopped venturing out unless accompanied by my husband. But the isolating effect was wearing on me. Staying inside, I decided to stay focused on finishing my first book which I would release the following spring. However, those encounters often left me feeling on high alert, wondering how I would handle the next series of questions or when my children would be a wee bit older so we could venture into other spaces. The need to get myself out of the loop of thoughts of failure, frustration, and worry, and my body from aching after being triggered by these emotions, became paramount.

Having a practical set of ways to initiate the parasympathetic state of your nervous system is the first step in getting back into your body after moments of feeling triggered, ashamed, embarrassed or simply overwhelmed by the outside world's questions, assumptions, or projected unrealistic timelines for healing. It's the first step to actualizing the slowing down your postpartum body really needs. Only when you are calm and cleared can you begin to make peace with being in a season of major physical, mental, emotional, and spiritual transition, much like I was. While I am sure the women I met at the playground meant no harm, these daily activities only served as a constant reminder that perhaps I was doing something wrong by taking time off. You can learn, as I did, to avoid this cyclical dance of trying to keep things business-as-usual when in fact, they aren't. I was in a season of transition, and maybe you are too.

Moments and situations like these can cause your season of transformation to get stunted, as you get distracted by the uncertainty of it all. Instead of allowing yourself to get wrapped up in the future, which will make your progress with healing take longer, there are accessible methods you can use to bring your nervous system out of the hazardous state of sympathetic. You can tell you're in this state if your heart is racing and your hormones are emitting through your armpits the most horrid of scents (trust me, I had plenty of moments when deodorant couldn't help me no how), or the tightening of your chest or back makes you feel like you cannot take another second. In moments like these, I learned to turn to my breath.

Breathwork

You might not realize it, but every time you take a breath, you are bringing energy in the form of oxygen into every cell of your body, which is critical for healthy functioning. For starters, maintaining healthy blood sugar levels requires that your body receive the right amount of oxygen; your brain requires five times as much oxygen than the rest of your cells; your liver, which manages emotions like anger and frustration, begins to express depressed functioning when oxygen levels in the body decrease. This is all to say, not only is your breath essential to keeping you alive, but using it effectively positively impacts you and your process to wholeness in very specific ways. Beginning with restoring optimal flow of qi or energy to your organs, when we breathe both deeply and correctly, we are releasing pent up toxins in the body, as well as blockages caused by experiences like birth trauma. However, most of us are not taking deep breaths; we are not in a space of awareness around how we're breathing. When stressful moments arise, our breathing can become even more shallow. Deeply disconnected from the actual role each part of our anatomy plays, many of us haven't had the chance to fully connect with the anatomy around our breathing. Take a second to observe your own breathing right now. Is it shallow? Are you breathing really quickly? Are your shoulders stiff? Does it hurt? Did you just stop to catch it because I mentioned it? If so, that's okay, but I guarantee you'll take a lot more notice of your breathing once you've tried all three of the forms I'm going to share below.

While each type of breath is aimed at calming your nervous system, slowing your heart rate, and getting you back into your body, breathwork brings healing when you are relaxed. Your goal isn't to strain, stress, or frustrate yourself as you work your way through each type. Simply set the intention to flow and allow each type to support you depending on what's happening in the moment.

Diaphragmatic Breathing

Diaphragmatic or Yogic breath is the first type of breathing we'll discuss and its use is great for moments when panic sets in, when a conversation you've had like the ones I shared above triggers fear, or when you simply want to interrupt negative thought patterns. This type of breath is what I like to think of as the "beginner's breath," because it causes you to practice greater awareness around shallow breathing and actually connect with the diaphragm, which is where optimal breath begins. This type of breathing also allows for oxygenation of your cells—you might not realize, but fresh air really supports the nourishment of the cells and organs we talked about in chapter five. Taking these deep, cell-nourishing breaths will really support your liver qi, which means all those 500 functions it is responsible for will get the proper support.

To do this type of breathing for the first time, sitting or standing, I want you to gently close your eyes, place one hand over your rib cage, and slowly pull your breath all the way in via the nose. As you do so, you should feel your hand rising as air fills into your lungs to the bottom of the diaphragm. When you've reached a place of being comfortably full, and your belly is extended, gently release the air, again via the nose and all the way out until your hand is back to being flat on your chest. This action allows the diaphragm to be fully contracted. Do this for a count of five breaths. Gently in through the nose and gently out through the nose, quietly. Don't worry if your face makes a grimace when you first get started. It can honestly feel unnatural at first, to allow so much air into your body if you are used to shallow breathing, which most of us are.

Relaxing Breath

This second type of breath, also called the "4-7-8" works on a, you guessed it, 4-7-8 breath count. This type of breath works for situations of anxiety and stress because it calls your awareness to the counting as a way of becoming attuned with the breath, creating a calming flow over the body and allowing you to enter a parasympathetic state. This is great for times when you are having difficulty clearing your mind or staying calm. With the Relaxing Breath, you are still taking deep breaths to the diaphragm, but the focus isn't so much on filling up the lungs as it is on keeping you focused on the count as a means of slowing down completely.

To begin this type of breath, again sitting or standing, gently close your eyes and pull in your breath for a four count. You can use your fingers to steady the count when first trying it out. Once you've pulled in a fresh, deep breath, you'll want to hold that breath for a seven count. Again, you can use your fingers to steady the count. After the seven second hold, gently release for an eight count. Use your fingers for steadying. This breath also encourages the releasing of any stale air in the lungs. You can do this up to three to four times so as not to get dizzy if this is your first time engaging in deep breathing.

Anchoring Breath

This third and final type of breath is great for those who are particularly empathic or highly sensitive and you find it hard to collect yourself after exchanges that leave you feeling drained. It helps you to clear yourself and get grounded. This particular type of breath also includes deep, diaphragmatic breathing but on the exhale, you want to make the breath audible. I envision it sounding like a cold winter breeze. So again, gently close your eyes, sitting or standing, inhale a nice, deep breath to fill the lungs to the diaphragm and release through the mouth, making the loud airy sound.

Practicing these different types of breath regularly—but most specifically when facing an onset of emotional turbulence or even simple moments like trying to start your day peacefully—will support you mentally, physically, emotionally, and yes, spiritually.

This shift can occur with a consistency of just four intentional minutes daily. As you become more and more comfortable with tapping into your breath for support with navigating triggering or stressful moments, the body and the organs affected by the different emotional stress responses can begin to heal.

Another cause or trigger for having your nervous system shift from parasympathetic to sympathetic during those early seasons of postpartum recovery, I discovered, is deeper ingrained layers of perfectionism that were groomed over time by this particular need to keep up. This country's economy , and the way it has influenced our generation's collective subconscious with its need to constantly produce content to stay afloat, only ramps up the need to multitask and create more lists for effectiveness. The problem is that all of this productivity doesn't make space for the changes a "slowness in pace" requires. Slowing down and not acting from a hypervigilant space is the most foundational way to allow the healing and change that you are yearning for. But there's something about the way we treat motherhood, especially as millennials, that makes it seem like this enormously life-altering responsibility and need for slowness is no more significant than a running title on your LinkedIn profile or Instagram bio. It's there, but shouldn't be a cause for distraction; it's just something we tack on while we strive to keep going, and by going I mean "after the dream." If you come from the world of academia like I do, your "dream" might entail becoming a professor, becoming an entrepreneur with multiple streams of income, not having a traditional 9-to-5 career, all goals research highlights as characteristic to us.

In my case, in 2016 before having my son, the dream was to get situated in my new career and role as a full-time school counselor. It's what I had fought tooth and nail for when I graduated from my master's program, and even though the gestational illnesses somewhat derailed me from being able to celebrate, my dream was to heal and get back to it. I had students to reconnect with and help grow. My first head-on collision with needing to make space for rest came when I had to accept two things that were very unexpected: one, my position was no longer open; and two, my body was not healing quick enough. And by quick enough, I mean there was no way on God's anointed Earth I was going to be able to throw on some heels and run up and down anybody's stairs the way the position required. By the May after I had given birth, I could barely touch my abdomen. My hair was steadily falling out. A bottom tooth had chipped out. But despite all these physical signs, I still fought to apply to other positions, unable to relinquish my grip on "the dream." I kept thinking this whole thing was my fault! I was supposed to be able to go back to work. I got even more angry because deep down inside, I knew it really wasn't my fault, but I had nowhere tangible to put this information. I just knew, based on all the rapid-fire decisions being made around my need to stay home, that I was used to being productive and on assignment. It was a fundamental part of my identity and, being the daughter of immigrants, it was doubly reinforced. From a socially subtle place, the message from the women before us was that going back to work made sense. I learned that summer of 2017 just how emotionally painful the effects of this surgery were and that I couldn't just barrel through the way I was used to doing.

On one occasion, one spring afternoon as my first book tour was beginning to settle down, I picked up the phone and dialed up a woman with whom I'd begun somewhat of a mentor/mentee relationship with. I had finally put the kids down for a nap and was free to discuss the future projects we had agreed to serve as accountability partners for. Up until that point, I had never taken the time to truly express to anyone outside my practitioner the difficulties I was experiencing around transitioning into a full-time stay at home mom. But on this particular afternoon, we were casually discussing daily routines and habits when I started lamenting about how difficult it was to keep a practical routine with my then two-year-old and one-year-old. I gently eased into sharing how frustrated I felt with not being able to get all the things on my to-do list done. There was a small pause before she replied that I simply "needed more discipline," that there was a friend she had who had five kids and could also serve as a mentor. This mother of five could share with me how she was able to "manage it all." What started off as an exciting exchange came to a screeching halt because in that moment, I felt myself break out into a humiliating sweat, the type of sweat that made me want to run and take a quick shower to escape the heat that was rising all over. It was clear a need for flexibility wasn't being perceived as that, but rather an inability to adapt.

The other socially subtle message women struggle with is this very pervasive belief, especially within communities of faith, is that with God all things are possible, that all you need to do is really "get it together and pray about it." For this person and many like her, the expression of being unable to accomplish goal-orienting tasks implies that you are not exercising your faith properly, that an element of your daily structure was out of alignment. However, you can be a woman of faith and still be faced with seasons of limitation. You can have faith in God, knowing He will grant you the strength, wisdom, and clarity to not only cast new visions and dreams, but to carry them out, but He will also see you through times of limitation. What this season was teaching me and maybe you, is that these limitations don't make you a bad mom or believer. It is a popular default in our current culture, even in the midst of a pandemic, to barrel through difficulty to accomplish a thing—or many things if you're a millennial mom. The problem is that mothers of a particular generation never learned that certain seasons of our lives, especially if entered into haphazardly, can be excruciatingly difficult. We simply don't want to hear that, and research confers this as a truth. We want to get through a thing as quickly as possible and generations ahead of us do a number on reinforcing this message that you can and should be able to "just do it." This makes it very difficult to admit when you cannot "just do it." This is why the comment from the mentor I mentioned, cut so deeply. Having no intimate understanding about the stage I was in, despite my being very active on a book tour, she just assumed it was something I wasn't mastering. She was right. I still hadn't mastered the stage of rest I truly needed. And to get there, two more holistic tools would be added to my wellness plan.

Originally developed and used in traditional Chinese medicine, Japanese massage, qigong, and yoga for thousands of years, tapping works through finger-tip tapping of acupuncture points on the body. In the West, it became known as Emotional Freedom Technique or EFT, thanks to Stanford University engineer Gary Craig. Craig, who is responsible for the modality being accepted as an evidence-based method for alleviating symptoms of post traumatic stress and anxiety, simplified it and proved its connection between cognitive therapy and acupressure. EFT is essentially a technique that works by dissolving pain along acupressure points attached to bigger umbrella emotions such as grief, anger, sadness, or fear. This can be linked to why I shared, back in chapter six, the importance of understanding how our emotions and feelings are linked to our organs and the flow of energy. Tapping works through light tapping on specific meridian points (a detailed image of these points can be found at the back of this book) and emotional blockages impacting those meridians are cleared from your subtle energy field. More specifically, for flashbacks and moments of panic, sometimes the more destabilizing effects of post traumatic stress, you can use tapping to release the stress you're feeling in the moment. Start by focusing on the event of the birth itself, while you tap as part of step one. For overall physical, emotional, and spiritual health being out of balance from triggers like the conversation I mentioned, I'm going to share some sample reminder phrases to guide you through. Feel free to use whichever phrases resonate with you most.

Starting EFT

Step 1: Identify the emotion you'd like to tap out. Is it anger, sadness, fear, anxiousness, worry, disappointment, resentment? Hold your active memory, emotion, or select a sample reminder phrase below. Identify from a scale of 1-10 the intensity of the feeling and where the stress is radiating most.

Sample Reminder Phrases

"Even though I am afraid to talk about my c-section experience, I deeply and truly and sincerely accept myself." (kidney/bladder)

"Even though I feel angry about my professional situation abruptly changing, I deeply and truly and sincerely accept myself." (Liver)

"Even though I can't let go of blaming myself for how my birth went, I deeply and truly and sincerely accept myself." (Colon/ Large Intestine)

[7] Church D, Stapleton P, Vasudevan A, O'Keefe T. Clinical EFT as an evidence-based practice for the treatment of psychological and physiological conditions: A systematic review. Front Psychol. 2022 Nov 10;13:951451. doi: 10.3389/fpsyg.2022.951451. PMID: 36438382; PMCID: PMC9692186.

"Even though I am angry for being judged for not suing my doctor, I deeply and truly and sincerely accept myself." (Liver)

"Even though I am overwhelmed from betrayal, I deeply and truly and sincerely accept myself." (Lungs)

"Even though I am worried about the direction of my future, I deeply and truly and sincerely accept myself." (Spleen)

"Even though I am overwhelmed by my new daily routine, I deeply and truly and sincerely accept myself." (Heart)

"Even though I feel vulnerable to the questions and judgments of others, I deeply and truly and sincerely accept myself." (Small Intestine)

Step 2: As you focus on the memory, begin to gently tap with your fingertips four to seven times, at the following meridian location points, in this particular order:

- Top & center of your head

- Between your eyebrows

- Outside of your eye (corner crease)

- Under the same eye

- Under your nose

- On your chin

- On your collarbone

- And finally, under your arm, right below your armpit

If you are using a reminder phrase, speak the phrase aloud as you tap the points.This will look like tapping the first point and saying aloud, "Even though I feel vulnerable to the questions and judgments of others, I deeply, and truly, and sincerely accept myself."Continue tapping the ordered points while speaking the phrase aloud. You can absolutely place the book down and give it a try here before continuing so as not to feel overwhelmed on your first try. If you're getting the hang of it, move on to step three.

Step 3: Continuing to hold the memory or speaking your phrase, you can begin to karate chop, which looks like taking the area of your pinky down to the bottom of your palm and karate chopping it into the space between your free hand's index and thumb. Karate chop for up to four to seven times.

Step 4: Stop and take notice of how the intensity behind the sensations linked to the memory or emotion behind your reminder phrase has shifted. On a scale of 1-10, give yourself a number. If you are feeling completely at a 1, you can stop. If not, return to step one and repeat the process until you find yourself at a more manageable number.

Aromatherapy

The final aspect of bringing your nervous system into a more parasympathetic state involves the use of essential oils or what is formally known as Aromatherapy, as we discussed in chapter four. While I know this ancient practice of using the aromatic, chemical compounds of plants and their various parts to shift emotions via the limbic system has become synonymous with multi-level marketing companies, using essential oils will always be about the noninvasive approach to supporting many of the body's systems and functions, particularly as they relate to mood improvement. Long before corporate establishments made essential oils popular again in the West, ancient peoples were using them to support wellness. As mentioned in chapter four, different oils are extracted from these different parts, including stem, flower, and petals, to create different effects. Through both inhalation and topical application, you can begin to experience the positive effects of their compositions almost immediately. For example, an oil that would be considered a grounding oil, such as cedarwood or vetiver, would come from the stem of the plant and could be used during times of extreme stress or a need to feel steady. Whereas for brighter scents like bergamot or rose, extraction would come from the petals of the flower and can be used when feelings of insecurity or low self-worth seek to overwhelm you. Each serves a unique purpose in creating a non-invasive way of supporting you and the key to seeing shifts is to work with them consistently. Let's explore the usage types.

Inhalation Method

When you inhale an essential oil, either by placing a few drops in your bare hands, using a roller stick inserted directly in the nostril, or locally in a room diffuser, the scent goes up your nose to the olfactory nerve, which directly corresponds with your sense of smell. This sense of smell directly impacts a part of your brain called the limbic system. The same way the scent of a certain fragrance can bring back thoughts of your favorite place to eat or that romantic first date, a certain smell can bring into remembrance aspects of your traumatic birth. From the smell of the food you ate during your stay, to the smell of the hospital room, to the fragrance your OBGYN wears, scents can act as triggers. Your sense of smell is directly linked to your memory bank, through your limbic system, which regulates your autonomic nervous system function. This controls unconscious functions like heart rate, breathing, pain and of course, emotions.

When you are working to activate a parasympathetic state, using this sense can positively impact your Limbic system. Inhaling or diffusing certain oils can expel certain negative emotions while stimulating more positive ones. For example, wild orange was the daily hug I never knew I would need. Diffusing it daily, in either the kitchen or my bedroom upon waking, helped me to feel abundant when I was a newly stay-at-home mom with two babies under two. Everyone around me was working outside the home, and full-time. Having this oil's fragrance permeating the air supported my entering a parasympathetic state because I was able to settle down into being open and optimistic; the essential oil's scent helped me to release the crippling fear of being alone with my kids for the first time, ever. This can be directly correlated with supporting the healthy flow of qi through the kidney and bladder meridians, as well as the amygdala in the brain which all govern the emotion of fear.

Not being wound up in fear eased my frustration from no longer being able to work outside my home. Like me, you might be emotionally torn between where you thought you were going and where your healing journey is actually taking you. It can feel like absolute hell on Earth to be pulled in such opposing directions, and then being led to feel like you have to suppress it all for fear of bearing the label of ungrateful, unstable, or depressed. Depending on where you live and the social construct of what race you are, these emotional descriptions can mean tons of different things. As a Black mother, who has a background in counseling, I struggled because I knew I was not downright depressed in the clinical, cut and dry fashion. I knew there were other things going on in my physical body that were causing me to feel the roller coaster emotions I was feeling. Put that into the context of what Sweeney & Meyers highlight in the Coping Self model as being affected by our living environments, and you have an added layer of fear. This season definitely exposed me to some very real limitations that mothers everywhere face when it comes to becoming whole again. Not being able to speak about what is really wrong emotionally also plays a role in the voice or throat chakra becoming unbalanced. We do not want people in our personal business, especially during this heightened time of technological overexposure. However, we find ourselves lashing out, quite critically, at others online and in our personal lives.

Initiating rest through the inhalation method with an oil like wild orange also helped to soothe these frustrations, by supporting what I've mentioned earlier as the liver and gallbladder meridians. The liver and gallbladder are two organs that play a critical role in the digestive process, but they also play a pivotal role in how our emotions are expressed, especially the emotion of anger. Energetically, the liver houses the psyche or emotion of anger and when we are either repressing, suppressing, or overexpressing this emotion the body can be thrown out of balance. This can manifest as headaches, shoulder pain, and even excessive belching. When our environments activate a state of rest within us, these emotions get the opportunity to dissipate as the balance of chi is restored and the body is brought back into a state of balance. This is exactly what happened for me as I began to work with this oil over the course of a few months, until I became more and more at ease with my role as a full-time stay-at-home mom and author. The nagging pain from all the frustration, trapped in my right shoulder blade, eventually began to dissipate. If you're wondering if wild orange is the only essential oil you can work with to cultivate a state of rest, I want you to know it is not and I will share a list of others, along with what emotions they promote via their properties and what emotions they support the body in releasing. But first, let's explore the secondary form of use, which is topical application.

Topical Method

With the inhalation method of working with essential oils, you can activate rest by smelling the oils to support the organs of the body under the stress of a particular emotion. However, with the topical method, you are applying the essential oils, appropriately diluted, to your skin, which is your biggest organ. Whether you realize it or not, everything you put on your skin is going directly through the epidermis and is being absorbed in the bloodstream, impacting, you guessed it, different organs and systems of your body. Therefore, with this method, you are diluting your essential oils in a carrier oil of your choice, and then applying it to different areas of the body to stimulate the properties of the essential oil in your body. For example, if you are feeling unable to connect with your c-section scar, as I was unable to even touch my scar for many months during the first year of postpartum, applying oils made for expelling apathy and fear, inviting courage and connection would be very beneficial. In the context of activating rest for your nervous system, applying oils that are calming, grounding and stabilizing to the soles of your feet and along your spine, is a safe and non-invasive approach to feeling better and more capable.

Essential Oils for Grounding and Activating REST in the Body

Dilution all depends on the size of your carrier bottle, but a 2-4% dilution rate is pretty standard. This involves using six to nine drops of essential oil to two teaspoons of carrier oil.

1. Cedarwood (Cedrus atlantica)

- Negative emotions: lonely, anti-social, disconnected
- Positive emotions inspired: supported, sociable

2. Vetiver (Vetiveria zizanoides)

- Negative emotions: scattered, stressed, crisis, ungrounded
- Positive emotions inspired: present, emotionally aware, grounded

3. Wild Orange/Orange (Citrus sinensis)

- Negative emotions: discouraged, lack of energy, envious
- Positive emotions inspired: warm, abundant, optimistic

4. Frankincense (Boswellia serrata)

- Negative emotions: spiritually disconnected/dark, abandoned, deceived
- Positive emotions inspired: wisdom, discerning, spiritually connected, protected

5. Roman Chamomile (Anthemus nobilis)

- Negative emotions: discouraged, frustrated, unsettled
- Positive emotions inspired: relaxed, peaceful, guided

6. Myrrh (Commiphora myrrha)

- Negative emotions: neglected, unsafe, distrusting, spiritual disconnection (maternal energy)
- Positive emotions inspired: nurtured, trusting, bonding, grounded, secure

7. Lavender (Lavandula augustifolia)

- Negative emotions: blocked in communication, feeling unseen, tense

- Positive emotions inspired: calm, expressive, self-aware, peaceful mind

8. Patchouli (Pogostemon cablin)

- Negative emotions: body shame, ungrounded, body tension, disconnection from body

- Positive emotions inspired: grounded, confident, body acceptance, balanced, stable

9. Peppermint (Mentha piperita)- not for use if breast-feeding

- Negative emotions: unbearable pain, intense despair, heavy hearted

- Positive emotions inspired: optimistic, relieved, strengthened

Much like the reminder phrases from the EFT Tapping, you can use affirmative statements as a compliment to inhaling or applying the essential oils. Not only does this help to activate the qualities of the oils themselves by linking the scent to the words being logged into your memory at the time of usage, but positive affirmations are also scientifically proven to change your subconscious pattern of thinking. Here are some unique affirmations I have created just for you.

7 AFFIRMATIONS FOR ACTIVATED SUPPORT DURING TOPICAL APPLICATION:

- "Where I am currently matters. I am grounded, rooted, and divinely supported."

- "I am capable of creating my own way. I am capable of having clarity in the direction of my future and my ability to Mother my children. I have purpose in my Mothering abilities."

- "I am worthy of transformation. I am worthy of a new identity. I have purpose in my new life. I am securely grounded and without resentment."

- "I am allowed to flow in abundance and grace. I am allowed to peacefully change and adapt to my circumstances."

- "I am worthy of receiving rest. I am worthy of receiving recuperation. I am worthy of asking for the help I need to receive the support to rest. I am capable of receiving new wind."

- "I am connected to the Divine Father. I am connected to the support of the Divine Mother. I am grounded in the direction my faith wants to grow. I surrender to the lessons my faith is teaching me."

- "I am able to establish new boundaries in my relation to myself and others. My heart is lifted from the hardening plaque of pain."

While I am sure the women I met at the playground or the mentor-friend I shared details with meant no harm, these normalized daily activities only served as a constant reminder that some think that mothers who do decide to take "more time" to heal are doing something wrong. Having the internal courage to defend your stance might not be readily available to you right now, while you learn to redefine what rest means for you. However, you can learn, as I did, to avoid this cyclical dance of guilt and shame in trying to keep things business as usual when in fact, they might not be. Putting in place these rituals of breathing more deeply, rewiring the way you speak to your rising fears, and using aromatherapy to adorn your body while shifting your daily mood into practice, is a loving way to invite peace and clarity to your postpartum journey. A loving way to begin the process of reclaiming your voice from the pain of your traumatic c-section experience.

Chapter 7

Replenish

The purpose of the Replenish chapter is to talk about how disconnected we can become from our physical bodies and how to eat appropriately based on the needs of different organs and body systems in order to heal. Recovering physically from the trauma of an unplanned, preventable, or even near-death c-section is often centered on the external experience more than the internal. What I mean by that is most c-section recovery books speak to us in a bit of a superficial way, if you will. I believe their concern is more fixated on the way we need to look rather than the way we want to feel or dare I say, need to feel, which is grounded, balanced, and full. Not only are we in need of healing tissue impacted by a several layered incision, but we are in need of rebalancing the communication between our gut and our brain. We need to protect neurotransmitters from inflammation, which can interfere with the effectiveness of communication, often determining our emotional health. But their focus remains on repairing the functioning aspects of our lives, i.e. we're told how to work through physical disruptions around abdominal diastasis. We're told not to do any heavy lifting, to avoid going up and down stairs too early, and we're even given a relatively universal approach to when it's safe (I'm not sure by whose vaginal measuring metrics) to reengage in sexual intercourse. I almost screamed when I read that, based on a national study's results, on average, couples resume intercourse seven weeks postpartum. I did a double take when I read, "Women who had c-sections resumed intercourse slightly sooner than those who'd given birth vaginally. That makes sense when you consider that a cesarean delivery doesn't leave you with the same sensitivity as a woman who delivers vaginally." I did a double-take because having had both forms of delivery, I can confirm sex after a c-section is nowhere near easier than sex post vaginal delivery. A survey conducted amongst my podcast listeners yielded a very different set of results from the national average, with an average of 12 weeks minimum being the waiting time and most directly related to the emotion of fear, specifically around the stitches "tearing" or "completely ripping."

I remember the first time I actually touched my physical scar. I spent almost three months unable to touch my scar, or even to acknowledge its literal presence. Thankfully, my husband was the type to truly care for me, pulling back the gauze daily to clean the scar. Laying me flat on my back on our living room carpet to gently cleanse the area, I was in too much pain to really be able to do it myself and I would break out into tears. I still couldn't believe it was there. It was one thing to recognize that I'd had the surgery, but it was another to begin reconnecting to my physical body. I felt for those first six months like I was a foreigner in my own skin. As a former athlete, having played every single sport except for football, hockey, and tennis, I was used to running, squatting, lifting weights, and otherwise being physical without having to think much about it. After the surgery, I developed a paralyzing fear of moving too much. I often felt like the wrong move would send my stitches flying in separation. It was just all too much. I resolved to wearing big sweatpants that could go up and down without much hassle, loose robes, oversized sweaters—anything to just keep me from bumping into my newly formed abdomen. I also learned wearing my beloved high heels was an absolute no-no. My frame felt so unsupported and ached after just a few hours of wearing them. Having foundational knowledge in naturopathy, I knew my body was experiencing or rather reacting to not just an abdominal surgery, but an overall structural change.

While I managed to shed much of the weight I gained during pregnancy through breastfeeding, the effects of the medication and the overall stress of the changes I was facing began to wear me down. One night, while selecting pictures for an episode of my podcast, I grabbed the rest of a sandwich I'd been meaning to finish. I took a hearty bite when I could feel something break. I actually couldn't take another bite, too full of fear that I'd choke on broken tooth pieces. I couldn't believe it, but I would later learn the tooth that broke was directly related to meridian lines 18 and 19. These lines are related to grief, sadness, and feeling imprisoned. To be quite honest, I was in disbelief and denial much of the time, believing my ever and always resilient self could simply power through this experience. I wasn't prepared for needing to make the tough decision of not going back to my full-time position. Then came the decision to cut off all my hair, from lion-mane, shoulder-length to an afro bordering a curly high top, then eventually a near cesar. So much of it was falling out beyond the typical postpartum shedding that I'd had it with trying to hold on.

I felt bold for doing it, cutting off section by section with a barber's scissor, while my husband tried to set a mood of "freedom" as he blasted songs by Anita Baker, Toni Braxton, and Sade, while holding a glass of wine on standby in case I got stuck along the way. I didn't get stuck, but I struggled with feeling beautiful. I came face to face with my vanity and struggled with having to let go of one more thing that I really loved about myself, my hair. I'm not makeup savvy, or what some would call high maintenance in my femininity, but my hair was the expression of my femininity. Its length and thickness made up for all the other things I wasn't interested in doing to be "pretty." Eventually, after a true cut from my husband's longtime barber-friend, I would begin to fall in love with who I was becoming. But that would not come without needing to learn how to build a relationship of compassion and nourishment with my physical body.

When you experience a traumatic c-section, not only are you navigating the healing of tissue being cut through on a very visceral level, but the organs untouched by surgery, touched by the memories and feelings left behind. Often when we hear about c-section recovery, we are given ways on how to achieve a beautiful snap-back shape; however, if you're the type of person who has never had a healthy relationship with food or believed diets were something you hopped on when you needed a certain result, then thinking about your snap-back body can feel beyond discouraging. Remember Marie, who felt guilt-ridden over her daughter's early birth? Her early postpartum journey is a perfect example of this. Determined to shed the weight she'd gained during this pregnancy, she worked to change her caloric intake over and over, and even sought to incorporate physical activity through the use of an indoor elliptical. She was taking very proactive steps to shed the weight; however, her struggles can speak to a real disconnect mothers experience between what we eat and why we're eating. We're not eating a certain way because we've made the connection to healing properties and feeling good, but we're often only focusing on achieving a specific weight while the emotional upsets from the birth are still there just below the surface.

But here's where I would like to draw your attention to how much the way you reorganize your understanding of the role of food and daily nourishment, along with other foundational lifestyle practices applied in a practical way, can help you cultivate not only a physically healthier version of yourself, but one that is also vibrant and emotionally grounded. This can be beneficial even beyond your first year postpartum.

What We Learned About Digestion

Yes, we are starting with the source or mechanics of how we eat. Not the how as in choices, but the actual process of how we engage with our meals. Did you know the process of how your body absorbs all those nutrients begins the minute you put food in your mouth? We might have learned about the body back in high school, but not necessarily in a way that teaches us how to form healthy connections with how we engage with our meals. Advertising basically tells us our country runs on coffee brands and the pun might as well be intended. We are all running, talking, scrolling, driving, streaming, and email corresponding while eating. The busyness of daily life takes over with schedules and to-do lists, and our often good intentions around eating healthily get thrown out the window. Emotions like anger, shock, frustration, or even sadness start to unconsciously play a part in our digestion process and before we know it, we're finding our appetites diminished or we're skipping meals altogether. When it comes to putting the nourishment back into our nutritional practices, we have to start with food as we experience it, creating an hospitable environment for the process.

Mastication

The process of chewing food completely, where enzymatic juices are released and prepare the food to go down your esophagus and into the stomach, is called mastication. Unfortunately, in today's culture and especially as mothers, the idea of chewing your food thoroughly to the point of mush for absorption is incredulous. We don't talk about this process because we believe digestion starts in the stomach and really only matters if we notice something is wrong, like heartburn or indigestion. We also treat eating to be nourished as somewhat of a luxury instead of the process that leads to healthfulness. And then there's the thing around time. I know as you're reading this, you might have already grimaced, thinking, "who has the time?" And trust me, I hear you, but it really just takes some shifting of your mindset around why we really eat and how ineffective it will be to your healing if you're not consciously engaging with the food or drink the minute it goes in your mouth. For starters, for your next meal or even snack, I want you to try to refrain from talking while you chew. Consciously take your time with chewing your food thoroughly. If you're used to talking on the phone, thinking it's your only free time to connect with friends or call back that aunt you've been meaning to, be a bit selfish and stay focused on the food. How does it taste? Do you notice yourself feeling fuller faster? After you've eaten, do you feel bloated or do you feel satisfied? Now begin practicing this at every meal until it feels second nature. This subtle change and these simple observations can really help you make a connection with the process that begins sending nutrients to the organs connected to your healing.

The digestive process has been commonly taught to us through biology classes: it begins when food goes down the esophagus to the stomach and enzymatic juices are released from the pancreas and liver. The food, now chyme, makes its way to the small intestine to synthesize, assimilate, and absorb nutrients the body needs to function optimally. Once all of that has happened, whatever is left gets transported to the large intestines where water is absorbed into the system, and the left over or undigested food becomes fecal matter and is excreted through the anus and through the rectum.

Sounds pretty straightforward right? Well, yes, in its optimal state of functioning, it is both simple and pretty complex because the state of your nervous system, as we briefly explored in chapter one, also determines how well these processes occur. For example, I just mentioned one of the biggest problems we as mothers in the West face is the constant running while eating, or being distracted while eating. Under these circumstances, the autonomic nervous system, which controls your sympathetic (flight or fright/voluntary system function) and parasympathetic (rest and digest/ involuntary function), is switched to sympathetic. When this happens, much of your system is in an emotionally heightened, charged state. This impacts every single one of your digestive organs' ability to break down, assimilate, and synthesize the nutrients you need to be optimally well. C-section births, while sometimes a life-saving intervention, can deeply impact the digestive system if not healed from properly. This is because a lot of inflammation can occur, hampering vital communication between the gut and the brain—where the nutrients you need for emotional healing are circulated. So when you eat, it's important to remember that it's not all about eating for calories to look better, but nourishing yourself correctly to literally feel better, and this again starts with the how of it all. Unfortunately, because treating ourselves like rundown robots seems normal, this key piece of knowledge and education is gone and it is assumed that when a mother is unable to shake symptoms of post-traumatic stress, she is going in a downward spiral and is now an automatic candidate for a clinical diagnosis. While I am not downplaying the severity of any clinical diagnosis by any means, I am saying this downward spiral doesn't always have to happen if we are aware that when nutrients aren't properly and adequately absorbed by the system, organs linked to our emotions cannot be adequately nourished. From a prevention-based approach, let's go a little deeper into this digestive process, emotionally, and understand what happens and what can go wrong.

What Pain Meds & Other Chemical Substances Do to Gut Lining

Healing from a c-section isn't just about having your reproductive system and muscles heal from abdominal surgery; your digestive tract will also need support as your gut flora can get knocked out of balance thanks to the presence of prescribed pain medication. Continued use of these drugs can also cause the lining of the small intestine, which is designed to filter harmful substances, bad bacteria, and undigested food out from the bloodstream, to weaken. This can lead to what we now call "leaky gut syndrome," which also interrupts your digestive system's ability to properly distribute nutrients to the bloodstream. While we know how beneficial and even necessary it is to have pain relief, it is important to know that balanced bacteria in both your small and large intestines is what supports your entire body from developing infections along your postpartum journey. Substances such as anesthesia (used during the surgery), narcotics (Percocet and codeine), blood pressure medication (if you were pre-eclamptic), acetaminophen, antibiotics, antidepressants, and NSAIDs (nonsteroidal anti-inflammatory drugs) all impact good bacteria in different ways, including affecting the production of vitamin B12, which is responsible for the building, repairing, and detoxifying of cells during energy production and healthy immune system function. In order to restore the flora that has been harmed and properly nourish whatever good bacteria you have left, both probiotics and prebiotics can be of great help.

As we've just explored the process that begins digestion, there can be confusion around what prebiotics and probiotics are, what they do, and whether or not both are needed. Prebiotics are dietary fiber and food constituents that act as a foundational support to good bacteria in your gut. They are carbohydrates that allow good bacteria in your gut to flourish. One example and important prebiotic is Inulin and it can be found in Dandelion root, Chicory root, and Artichoke. Beans, legumes, berries, and greens like arugula, bok choy, and kale are also great prebiotics. Probiotics, on the other hand, are actually live organisms that are good bacteria taken in the form of supplements. They match what can already be found in your body. The most popular strain is L.acidophilus, however this is just one of six strains that are considered "resident strains," which are expected to be part of your intestinal microbiome. The other six are as follows: Lactobacillus salivarius, Bifidobacteria bifidum, Bifidobacteria infantis, Bifidobacteria logom, Streptococcus faecalis, and Streptococcus faecium.

Both prebiotics and probiotics should be taken at the start of every meal, however, renowned chiropractor Dr. Susan Levy recommends having a morning formulated and an evening formulated probiotic. While prebiotics, as mentioned, are available in certain foods, probiotics can be found in liquid form, capsules, powder and even pearl forms from holistic health or natural health stores and health food locations. We all could benefit from incorporating these two tools to support the absorption properties of the digestive tract, but especially when healing from c-section birth trauma. In that case, when absorption can be negatively impacted, they will make it much easier to see the effects of working with your meridian pairs as a means to balancing your emotional health. Now let's look at what nourishment for each meridian pair looks like.

The Stomach/Spleen

As we explored in chapter one, the stomach and the spleen meridians share the same element of Earth energy and can be linked to the emotions of worry and anxiety. It is no secret that when you're overcome by thoughts of whether you'll get rehired at work (worry) or if people will look at you funny for deciding to give up work outside the home altogether (anxiety), even if you've chewed your food thoroughly, this can result in stomachaches, indigestion, nausea, heartburn, belching, and even chronic diarrhea. As birth trauma can leave behind the emotional effects of hypervigilance, paying attention to the support of these two meridians can promote positive change. Supporting the spleen, which houses our thoughts and the quality of them in traditional Chinese medicine, through spleen supportive nutrients, oxygenated blood and energy needed to transform old red blood cells is available to support its functioning. The stomach, which the spleen is paired with, and your entire immune system, which also plays a vital role, all benefit.

Incorporating foods rich in vitamins C, B, and B complex is clutch. For vitamin C, foods include bell peppers, strawberries, broccoli, and leafy greens. Vitamin B complex can be found in liver, fish, poultry, and eggs; if you are vegetarian or vegan, you can consume beans and peas, dark leafy greens, and whole grain cereals. Minerals such as magnesium, potassium, iron, and copper are also essential to strengthening these organs for optimal functioning. You can find these nutrients in foods such as fish, nuts (think cashews, almonds, walnuts, pistachios), seeds (think flax, pumpkin, sunflower), and whole grains. Magnesium can also be taken, under your practitioner's supervision, in the form of a supplement either in liquid or capsule. The best form, as in easiest for the body to absorb, is magnesium citrate malate.

The Liver/Gallbladder

Governing emotions such as anger, frustration, resentment, rage and dissatisfaction, the liver and gallbladder pair is all about expansion and decision-making. When eyesight has become weakened or you feel pinching pain in your body, these are just a few physical tell-tale signs that this pair is in need of extra care. The rise of annoyance, inability to plan, depression, and feeling the need to self-isolate are signs this pair is losing qi and vitality. Understanding your need to slow down or altogether pivot with personal plans or even day-to-day activities, can help you connect with the liver and gallbladder meridians. Consuming vitamins such as vitamins A, B12, C, E, and niacin will work to support the pair's biochemical functioning. Minerals such as magnesium, potassium, iron and sodium are also essential to bringing back the nutritive qi it needs for optimal functioning. Foods that are supportive of this pair's healthy detox of toxins, bile formation, and blood filtration as part of its optimal functioning are raw leafy greens, avocado, whole grains, lamb, herring and eggs. Some herbs to consider are Alfalfa, Dandelion, Nettle, and Oatstraw.

Lungs/Large Intestines

Governing emotions such as grief, sadness, disappointment and shame, the lungs and large intestines meridian can express disharmony in several ways. From a weakened voice, shortened breath, coughing, and even upper respiratory tract infections to constipation, colitis and even irritable bowel syndrome, in extreme cases. While every pairing is important and essential to your overall health and wellness, this pair is extra special. This is because on the most visceral level, the c-section incision, as mentioned in chapter one, cuts through layers of tissue—including connective tissue, nerve, and of course muscle. When supporting the emotional balancing of this meridian, the foods consumed very much support the healing of scar tissue and ultimately your gut's communication with your brain via the gut-brain axis, which happens via the vagus nerve and autonomic nervous system pathways. Nourishing this meridian pair involves consumption of vitamins A, C, and E. All three vitamins work to speed up wound healing and tissue repair from the incision. Vitamin A also supports healthy mucous membranes throughout the digestive tract as well as increases your resistance to infection, something some mothers can experience post c-section surgery. Vitamin A can be found in dark leafy greens such as kale, orange or yellow vegetables and fruits, and in organ meats. Vitamin C, a powerful antioxidant and immune system booster, can be found in citrus fruits such as oranges, strawberries, broccoli, bell peppers, and leafy greens like spinach. And lastly, vitamin E, which is also a powerful antioxidant, keeps free radicals from damaging your cells and tissue while you heal. Vitamin E can be found in nuts, dark leafy greens, eggs, and avocados. Selenium, which acts as a perfect pairing to vitamin E's functioning, also supports the neutralization of certain chemical poisons like cadmium, mercury, and arsenic, which are sometimes inhaled or ingested. Foods such as asparagus, eggs, and mushrooms are a great source of nourishment for this particular vitamin.

Heart/Small Intestine

Governing emotions such as joy and sadness, courage and despair, love and hate, and the ability to receive, synthesize, integrate, and absorb information, the heart and small intestine meridians can signal their need to be balanced through several physical indications. For one, when these two are out of balance we can experience palpitations, constriction of blood vessels leading to elevated blood pressure, skin rashes, and sleep disturbances. Nourishing this meridian pair involves consumption of calcium, magnesium, potassium, and antioxidant Coenzyme or CoQ10. Calcium supports muscle contraction and heartbeat, and can be found in foods such as kelp, kale, collard greens, almonds, sesame seeds, goat milk, and broccoli. Magnesium maintains electrical charge in the cells of the body, such as heart cells, and can be found in foods such as wheat bran, wheat germ, coconut meat, brown rice, almonds, cashews, figs, apricots, and molasses. Potassium also protects the electrical charge of cells and when there is high potassium in the body, there is protection against things like elevated blood pressure. Potassium can be found in foods such as avocado, asparagus, carrots, lima beans, bananas, and cod.

Now, let's put into application this practice of eating using this meridian pair, organ-focused style of nourishment that can help you resolve some very real physical effects related to c-section delivery and healing.

Hair Loss

Connected to the energy of fear, or what traditional Chinese medicine classifies as Jing energy, hair loss can be directly related to the final meridian pair of importance- the kidney/bladder meridian pair. This pair encompasses the energetic function of your kidneys and adrenals. The emotional impact of a traumatic c-section directly influences the function of this meridian and when not properly addressed, causes physical effects such as fatigue, sleeplessness, dizziness, and even temperature dysregulation. This is why, when under extreme circumstances of stress, we can experience greater shedding or overall loss of hair, but rarely do we make the connection that fear plays a role in this. We often think it's just frustration or anger, which can promote stress, but fear can as well. Not to be confused with the natural aspects of the period of postpartum shedding, the restoration from hair loss can absolutely be supported by nutritionally supporting this organ's meridian. While the breathwork exercises from chapter six can support the release of these fear-linked emotions and get your nervous system into parasympathetic, which this meridian needs in order to function optimally, there are also ways to nutritionally support the return of your hair.

I am well aware that depending on your race and ethnic makeup, the way your hair grows back and the rate will definitely vary. Specifically, as a Black woman, I mentioned the experience of needing to cut off all of my remaining shoulder length hair down to what can be googled as a Cesar cut. Before your mouth drops in disbelief or fear that you have to do the exact same thing, I want to share that cutting your hair off and starting from scratch can be one of the most cathartic experiences in terms of letting go of the energy from the surgery. It's a great way to start fresh, but in case this sounds too extreme for you, nourishing the organs related to this particular issue is also a great place to start. Incorporating nutrients such as ashwagandha and alfalfa strengthen kidney functioning, along with magnesium and potassium. Potassium can be found in foods such as lean meats, avocados, citrus fruits, bananas, and potatoes. Magnesium can be found in dark leafy greens, nuts, seeds, and fish. While focusing on incorporating these foods, you can also reference the EFT protocol and tap out fear linked to starting your hair growth over, if necessary. Below, I am sharing one of my favorite juicing recipes that I used daily over the course of an entire year containing many of these nutrients for you to try out.

Dr. Laura's Juicing Recipe for Supporting Healthy Kidney Meridian

linked to Hair Growth (makes up to 16 oz.)

8 organic carrots

4 organic apples

1 bulk of organic celery

1 cup of organic kale

1 organic lime

1 teaspoon of turmeric

1 teaspoon of cayenne pepper

Vaginal Dryness, Decreased Sex Drive & Intimacy Change

While the decision to engage in sexual intercourse post-delivery truly depends on how your stitching is healing on the physical level, hormonal and emotional changes can deeply impact your ability to feel and be intimate with your spouse or partner. From feelings of impureness and guilt to shame, fear, or feeling undesirable, emotions can definitely impact your ability to experience pleasure post-birth. This can be a quiet, often shameful experience that comes in like a shocking wave for mothers because we're expected to know how to keep our sexy going, no matter what. However, re-establishing a healthy connection with your sense of intimacy and sexual health is important to your overall health. Incorporating foods and herbs that support the reproductive system, nervous system, and lymphatic system, specifically the spleen, which covers our thoughts and worries, is key. Herbs such as Skullcap, Vervain, and Passionflower are nervines and can support a more relaxed state, as the phases of sexual response for women begin from a balanced nervous system. Maca is an adaptogen and tonic that supports increasing sexual desire. However, if you know that you have iodine deficiency, it can mildly inhibit thyroid function, so it may be good to avoid. For vaginal dryness, it can be helpful to increase the intake of essential fatty acids from fish, including salmon and mackerel; flaxseeds and nuts, including walnuts; soybeans; and green leafy vegetables.

Muscle Spasms

As your abdominal muscles begin to heal, you might not expect it, but experiencing random moments of involuntary muscle cramping is common. While not serious, this often painful feeling, a stiff-like sensation on either side of your abdomen below your belly button can be attributed to several different factors: dehydration, over-exertion of these lower muscles, fatigue, and yes, a lack of nutrients in the system. I remember the first time this happened to me. I was around nine months postpartum and as I was turning to place my son into his crib, I felt a sudden tightening of my lower right abdomen. I literally froze as the pain was quick but very intense. It felt like I needed to just stay still and breathe for it to stop. While pelvic floor therapy and other forms of exercise are recommended for repairing these muscles impacted by c-section birth, we really need to keep in mind how essential rest and proper nourishment is to healing. Three key nutrients can be added to your daily nourishment practice are calcium, magnesium, and vitamin D.

The connection between the physical and emotional can be made through recognizing how the large intestine meridian corresponds to emotions like grief and the inability to let go, while the small intestine corresponds with the emotions of sadness. Therefore, when you take vitamins and minerals like calcium, magnesium, and vitamin D, you are not only supporting the repair on a physical level, but you are also mitigating the presence of negative emotions.

Dental/ Oral Health

Calcium, fluorine, zinc, and phosphorus are minerals the body requires and uses for the formation, fortification, and ultimately restoration of bones and teeth in the body. Calcium and phosphorus are responsible for bone and tooth formation. When you are pregnant, depending on the condition your body is in when you become pregnant, minerals can become depleted by the end of the pregnancy due to the needs of the growing baby who also absorbs these minerals. This is why prenatal vitamins and a focus on nutrition is emphasized. However, if the ability to absorb and maintain nutrients throughout the pregnancy cannot be achieved for whatever reasons, post-birth, the body can definitely find itself in a depleted state. After a c-section birth, in particular, a mineral like zinc will be required to properly heal. This is because minerals such as phosphorus, calcium, and zinc, in particular, are responsible for tissue growth and repair. This is a root cause as to why so many women, including myself, experience problems with their gums and teeth while healing from c-section delivery. This can include chipping, weakened enamels, and even complete breaking. To prevent demineralization of your bones and teeth while healing, it is important to incorporate foods such as freshwater fish, legumes, nuts, and whole grains to maintain a healthy amount of phosphorus. To prevent tooth decay, try to incorporate foods such as spinach and onions into your meals. To support wound healing, that being the c-section incision itself which requires minerals of the body, incorporating foods such as liver, herring, and eggs will be beneficial.

Other Lifestyle Foundations for Consideration

Sleep

Within the first year postpartum, creating a sleep routine can be extremely difficult. However, there are a few simple things you can do to promote a return to healthy sleep hygiene, even if it's a few hours at a time to start. Creatures of technology, it might come as second nature to have the phone near the bed or maybe in the bed with you, but that is the first place you want to start modifying. Exposure to Electromagnetic Fields, also known as EMFs, can cause your sleep to be disturbed. Turning it on airplane mode and placing it away from your bed is a great step. The type of lighting and atmosphere in your bedroom can cause your sleep to be disturbed as well. If you have blinds, make sure they are always shut before bed. If you have curtains, opt for dark shades if possible to keep all outside noise and light blocked out. Using aromatherapy combinations from chapter six in the form of diffusion greatly supports an environment for healthy sleep.

Hydration

Drink filtered water throughout the day. Drink half your water weight in ounces daily. If it is possible, add liquid chlorophyll to your drinking water as an excellent way to promote oxygenation in your blood and large intestine. Liquid chlorophyll can also support healing flora within the gut after taking medication from the c-section surgery. Soups, broths, and water fruits are also a great way to support hydration in the body.

Sunlight

Exposure to sunlight for just 20 minutes a day gives you healthful amounts of Vitamin D, supports a healthy circadian rhythm which allows you to get restful sleep, and has been clinically proven to support relief from nervousness by its positive impact on the pineal and pituitary glands. Whether you live in an apartment or a house, finding a way to get to a window, stoop, patio, porch, balcony, or even playground daily can support your physical body's need for solar nourishment.

Now that we have addressed how to use food and a mindset of nourishment to support our healing, I want to go back to the part where I mentioned learning to fall in love with my new haircut as part of the woman I was becoming. Remember when I said it didn't happen suddenly? That I had to learn how to bring my mind and my body back into connection by tempering my resilience with more compassion and grace? I also had to learn how to cast a new vision for myself—what I wanted to feel like, what I wanted to smell like, what I wanted my aura to resonate like. All of this is part of rebuilding your sense of self because it is incredibly easy to fall asleep at adorning yourself. For me, I fell asleep in the form of no longer buying any new clothes for myself because I just didn't think it was worth it. Knowing that I would no longer be waking up and getting dressed to go out to work, I found adorning myself to be pointless.

I had always practiced clean eating and was an advocate for eating well, but reorienting my mental and physical connection would mean needing to give resilience a break and taking on grace. Moving through the next stages of your healing journey would mean not just becoming reacquainted with the power of using wholesome, organic, and culturally relevant foods, but also casting a proper vision for how you want your body to look and feel.

The Power of Using Creativity to Cast a New Self-Image: Vision-Boarding

While many people might look at making vision boards as something of a simple pastime or tool for manifestation, causing you to frown on the practice or doubt its power in helping you to reclaim your narrative, creating vision boards is a great way to clear out your subconscious. What is it that you think about yourself? About yourself as a mother on this side of tragedy or as a result of experiencing the pain of a traumatic c-section? Do you now see yourself as weak? Do you now see yourself as disheveled and not worthy of building back your beauty? Is it possible you now see yourself as no longer creative or as a woman without sensuality or sex appeal? Do you see yourself as someone who should just shrink or hide away? If you answered 'yes' to any of the above, just know you are not alone. Know also that trauma has the ability to affect your imagination [Bessel, 16]. This is because when we experience trauma, on a physiological level the brain loses its flexibility. When that happens, you guessed it, your imagination is impacted. In the Sweeney Myers model, the Coping Self calls this "realistic beliefs."

When the initial haze of having just had a major c-section started to clear, the effects started to show up—like not being able to get back to work the way I thought I would, or the loss of my hair--I started to think and feel certain things about myself. I stopped getting pretty. I stopped buying new clothes to adorn myself. I started trying to overcompensate for the fact that I was transforming into a full-time stay at home mom. While I decided to finish and release my first book during this season, and looked beautiful during the tour season, I focused on the work of it all, not necessarily how I felt about myself. Internally, I wasn't feeling very sensual or like I should be shopping for my frame, which was struggling to keep weight up at the time. There came a point after the tour was over where I said to myself, "uh uh Laura, you gotta get it together honey!" I decided to go back to a favorite Biblical scripture that reads, "Write the vision and make it plain," which comes from Habakuk 2. I believe this is where the root of what we now hear in popular culture as, "write it down and watch it manifest." Well the same can be said for thinking about how you would like to look and feel while you are working to rebuild your strength and voice.

I decided to get going on a new vision for what I wanted to look like, how I wanted to feel and most importantly, what I thought about myself. I began the process of taking inventory around my realistic beliefs. Now you might be standing at the place where redefining yourself as a Matriarch is key to putting renewed wind beneath your wings. You would like to call in new energy and are not sure how to get started. Well, let me show you how!

First, I want to draw your attention to thinking about your favorite women in let's say entertainment or the arts. I want you to think for a minute what it is about these particular women you admire most. Is it their allure? The way they style their hair? Is it her choice of clothing? What do you admire most? Once you have figured out those important details, I would say you are going to need to invest in some tools. You'll need a pair of scissors, glue, scotch tape, cardboard or poster paper, and magazines. You might also want to print out or find in these magazines the faces of these women you admire. You are going to begin by clearing your subconscious mind—you can even say a small prayer for guidance—and begin to cut out words that inspire you about who you would like to become on this journey.

Let me give you an example. When I constructed my own Matriarch vision board, some of the words I felt called to cut out and paste were: calm, poised, graceful, feminine, authority, kind, adventurous, and of course, whole. Some of the women whose image I cut out to match what I felt I wanted to become were actresses Nicole Ari Parker and Nia Long. I connected with Nicole's upkeep of her beauty, health, and sensuality within her marriage to husband, Boris Kodjoe. When I look at a woman like her, I personally feel encouraged to keep up my essence as a woman. When I look at a woman like Nia Long, I am reminded of privacy. In the age of social media and constant exposure of what was once considered a private life, Nia reminds me and affirms my choice to keep a healthy set of boundaries around my private life. There might be other nameless women you come across as you are scouring images throughout magazines that you connect with. Perhaps it's the way the hair is styled or the clothing or the entire aesthetic that speaks to you. Cut them out and add them. The goal of this exercise is to dream, be inspired, and affirm your ability to recreate and essentially replenish yourself as a woman, and now, mother. The goal is to remove the shadow or newly formed identity of having experienced trauma and being pushed into silence. Use of this creative affirmation of your future self comes in handy whenever you find yourself shrinking, whenever you feel the weight of your birth narrative threatening to crush you and keep you from evolving. For me, the point of sharing this aspect of the method with you is to affirm that what you are feeling and have been experiencing is not abnormal, but that you can actively change your narrative in a very fun, simple manner. When you're done, and you feel you've gotten it all out, hang it somewhere you can see, daily. Maybe it's your bedroom door or the inside of your closet door; ready to see as you pick out your clothes for the day.

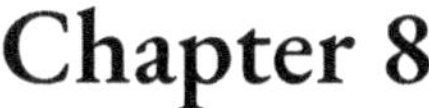

Chapter 8

Re-Evaluate

If the purpose of chapter six was to show you how being in a parasympathetic state would allow you to feel grounded in your body and chapter seven was about showing you how to use food as a tool for nourishing your physical body while also supporting you emotionally, then the purpose of this chapter is to help you with the last piece of what I believe supports the total realignment of calling back your voice from birth trauma, and that is acceptance around a change of will. The throat chakra, as we discussed in chapter five, is the energetic center of the body, which not only governs our ability to express ourselves in a balanced manner, but also regulates our ability to speak our truth, determines what truths we align ourselves with, and navigates personal will versus that of the Divine's will. Simply put, you might have had the perfect or "best laid" plans for what your life would look like after this birth. You might have made concrete preparations to take on a new role at work, resume a creative project, or resume a paused higher education program right after delivery, but the process of your healing– needing to slow down and literally catch your breath, the need to reestablish your relationship with mindful, intentional, nourished eating, and self redefinition—has taken over. Being able to speak about this birth, particularly as the haze of gratitude for being alive fades, in a manner that doesn't provoke feelings of resentment, betrayal, and anger, is the test around how well you are able to heal and truly move forward. Who and what do you sound like as a person who has accepted this birth despite the chaos it might have caused? This portion of the method is designed to help you sink your teeth patiently and discerningly into looking at not just the throat chakra, which governs timing in our lives, but all of your energetic centers. Here in this examination of these centers based on what they represent, you can make room to observe what messages they want to reveal to you about who you were before this birth and how you can use this information to spiritually reconstruct yourself in the after. You can think of this as a sort of spiritual surgery conducted simply yet powerfully with the tools of journaling, reflection, and contemplation—three things mothers of our generation are in dire need of reclaiming. With this very guided reflection aspect of the method, I sought to provide a way to help you safely ground your thoughts and feelings around these nuances as they begin to surface. Sometimes this surfacing happens in the earliest of days and sometimes it takes time to come through. However, looking at these thoughts and feelings in the context or container of your energy system- your chakras and what they represent in daily living- reevaluation of each center's representation can help you with the shift from woundedness to empowerment. What can you learn about yourself and your purpose? What can you release as well as invite in, once you understand how each energetic system has been impacted? Journaling is the first step.

While we might think of journaling as just a simple act of doodling our thoughts or writing down random emotions, according to studies conducted by the Positive Psychology Program, there are over 80 benefits to journaling, including the management of depression, anxiety, and general feelings of stress. Journaling reduces intrusive thoughts and avoidance symptoms post trauma. Writing down thoughts, emotions, or experiences can help us to work through our personal narratives, improve our working memory, and help us detect unhealthy patterns in our behavior. If you're navigating or have navigated symptoms of post traumatic stress, then journaling can be a source of safe processing, and the confronting of held back emotion related to the experience. In the approach of natural healthcare, journaling is encouraged as a meditative, stress reducing heart opener. It's a clear, free, and easy way to come into connection with who you are and the deeper contents of your soul. While I am highly aware this tool and technique may not be the first response for a mother who has already been diagnosed with a clinical condition as a result of this type of birth, it is supportive as a means of prevention. I also want to bring awareness to the fact that we don't live in those extremes—that unpacking through self-reflection the feelings of sadness, disappointment, and anger, does not automatically mean you are headed in the direction of a diagnosis. You are engaging in a practice of self-awareness, and by using the other parts of the method in combination with this, you can proactively work to heal your voice, and how you express your truth around the birth. So using this practice of journaling in the way I have combined it with looking at your chakra anatomy, gives you the structural focus that motherhood's overwhelm can sometimes rob us of unexpectedly.

The next aspect of Reevaluation is prayer and contemplation. Whether or not you consider yourself to be connected to a higher power, feelings of disconnection towards life itself after this type of experience can absolutely surface, giving way to persistent sadness, disinterest in daily activities, and loss of appetite. In traditional Naturopathy, this is referred to as shock and trauma, but more specifically as being disconnected from Source. Some circles may refer to this as experiencing a "dark night of the soul." This can lead to a feeling of purposelessness and without a sense of purpose in one's daily life, the will to survive can be weakened. While this is a vantage point that has not often been acknowledged in traditional mental healthcare, unless you are seen by a practitioner that has a faith-based dynamic to their philosophy of practice, in order to experience wholeness, there needs to be unification of the physical, mental, and spiritual self. Because in essence, this is who we are, not just as humans, but particularly as mothers. Experiencing trauma in the moment of bringing life into the world, especially via c-section birth trauma, can cause you to become extremely resentful in your connection to Source around what you thought your birth would be like, but also what postpartum life should look like. If you are a person of faith, you engage in faith-based practices, or you believe in prayer, shame and guilt might arise as you navigate questions like the following: "How could you let this happen to me, Lord?" or "I trusted God, now look what happened?" or "If God truly loved me, He wouldn't have let this happen to me. He knew I had plans?" Do any of these sound familiar?

Do you come from a family of origin where expressing oneself in this manner is frowned upon?

When there is an inability to reconnect to the foundation of your relationship to Source, feelings of sadness can persist, affecting not just the way you think, but your ability to find purpose in your motherhood. In my own journey, this showed up as needing to surrender perfectionism, the belief that I had to do everything in a certain way in order to regain productivity, and seeing how it was creating issues around my solar plexus and my adrenal health. In working with women like Diana, a mother who had three c-section births with two of them being traumatic in nature, and also being a sexual assault survivor, I could see the connection between her sacral chakra energy being off balance, painful periods, and her engaging in endless cycles of self-sabotage. Diana struggled to accept how despite being years well beyond these births, she was still being called to use her voice and experiences in a way that would support the collective in a major way. In working with her, it was clear how prayer was there, but contemplation through self-reflection based on the journaling practice was absent. She was resisting looking at herself and the messages of her energetic anatomy on paper. The subsequent alignment came once she committed to journaling and bringing those weaknesses back into her prayer life to be addressed. Understanding the difficulty that might be present when working to make all of these parts of yourself come together and the need for privacy around what the journaling portion might reveal for each subtle energy center, I've provided words of prayer for you. You can use them for moments or in this season when there is desire to connect to God, but you're simply out of words or not sure where to begin with reconnecting the dots. This is where all three- journaling, contemplation, and prayer come together, and I want to practice full transparency in sharing that my faith-based practice of prayer also involves scriptural verses, rooted in the Christian faith. However, with respect to all faiths, I simply invite you to integrate what resonates with your system of faith as you please. The ultimate goal is to help you reconnect with the actual presence, peace and purpose of the Divine in order to develop a renewed voice around your experience and your next chapter on this postpartum journey. So let's start by outlining what each chakra represents and the issues it prompts, followed by a series of guided questions to facilitate your personalized process. This will show up in the contemplation aspect. Using the Indivisible Self model mentioned back in chapter five, I am going to show you how you can ground these questions back into your everyday life, holistically, as you rebuild. This will serve as especially helpful to take notice of any patterns or blockages you've developed through your experience, even if you've passed the early postpartum stage of the first year.

The first chakra we will explore is the root chakra. Corresponding with your genitals, adrenal glands, some bladder and kidney functioning, and the skin, the root chakra is what keeps you grounded and connected to all the basic necessities in life, including food, shelter, your home and your tribe, also known as your family of origin. Muladhara, its original name in Sanskrit, the root chakra, is located at the base of your spine, connects the first three vertebrae and governs your emotional sense of safety and security in the physical world. When this chakra is disrupted or thrown off balance, the disharmony is manifested as feelings of anxiety, fear, sleeplessness, an inability to maintain healthy weight, hair loss, an inability to let things go, fears and even nightmares. Laziness, lethargy, and feelings of not belonging are expressions of underactivity. Here in this chakra, energetic and spiritual issues around what or where your place in the world exists, are up for examination.

The next chakra, represented by the color orange, is the sacral chakra. Governing the uterus and all aspects of the reproductive system from the region of the navel down to the pubic bone, Svadisthana governs parts of the adrenals, intestines, and neurotransmitters that determine emotional responses to stimuli. A chakra that is much about pleasure, personal joy, and cohesiveness with others, the sacral chakra is fundamentally about personal power, creativity, control and money. When out of balance, the manifestations are just the opposite. Fear of change, financial instability, sexual dysfunction, depression, self-sabotage, and addictions result from imbalance. The inability to creatively express yourself to others, or to connect emotionally with others, can attract partnerships and experiences that can actually oppress you and strip you of your sense of personal power. An example of this can be seen with Diana, the designer who had three c-sections. The first surgery's trauma only served to compact the emotional wounding of the sexual assault. Until she could acknowledge that she was constantly giving away her personal power to clients by not properly charging them for her creations or not suspending accounts when she wasn't paid at all, her throat chakra continued to remain totally unbalanced. She appeared to people as if she always was in a state of rage, yelling at people, speaking aggressively or completely out of turn. Not previously understanding the significance of her spiritual anatomy being disturbed, she would constantly feel embarrassed by her voice and unfit to accept that her higher purpose for experiencing the trauma was to help others through their own.

Next up is the solar plexus. The third chakra up, Manipura, as it is called, is represented by the color yellow and often reminds me of a beautiful, brazenly bold sunflower. This image is what led me to use the sunflower as the brand graphic for the podcast; it so deeply reminded me of the power of standing bright from a strong core, and that's what this chakra is all about. Governing many of the digestive organs including the liver, pancreas, gallbladder, stomach, and even parts of the urinary system, specifically the kidneys, the solar plexus physically governs the region between the navel and the base of the sternum. Emotionally, this chakra governs self-esteem, self-confidence, and self-worth. When in balance, this chakra, which represents our outward interaction with society, expresses itself as confidence in the contributions you make through the outward roles you take. When out of balance, this chakra manifests as being hyper-critical towards yourself and others, perfectionistic, unable to take personal responsibility, and unable to accept making mistakes. Imbalance in this chakra can lead to eating disorders, feelings of inferiority, and low self-esteem. An example of the solar plexus being out of balance can be seen through Melissa, who had the twins and felt hypercritical around herself and her weight early postpartum. Her desire to choose a holistic path to healing was not met with support by her family, and created a sense of fear around her ability to see losing weight all the way through naturally. This led her to creating dietary restrictions of all kinds as a means to try and lose the desired weight. However, her constant self-critiquing only made that process more scrutinizing.

Continuing to move upward, the fourth chakra, which is located at the center of the chest, is represented by the color green and is also known as Anahata. Anahata, or the heart chakra, governs the heart and circulatory system, lungs and respiratory system, breasts, thymus gland, and ribs. Emotionally, the heart chakra is indeed about love; however, it is also about forgiveness, compassion, and releasing the need to understand the "why" behind something's occurrence in our lives. The heart chakra is distinctively related to our ability to accept our emotional challenges while surrendering to the will of the Divine, the Creator. When in balance, the heart chakra manifests as being hopeful, loving, inspired, capable of trusting others, and accepting of love from the Divine. When out of balance, this chakra manifests as being jealous, bitter, hateful, unable to forgive yourself and others, and fearful of loneliness and commitment.

The sixth chakra, which follows the throat or fifth chakra covered in chapter five, is located between the brows. It is aptly called the brow chakra, but in Sanskrit it is called Ajna. Associated with the color purple and sometimes indigo, the brow chakra governs the pituitary and pineal glands, and the brain and neurological system. Emotionally, the brow chakra is about being able to "see clearly," and about having clean sight. And just what are you seeing? The choices regarding the path you've decided to take in life. The power to make rational and grounded choices towards your future is found here in this energetic center. Here we also face memories we hold in our mind's eye, our ability to practice detachment, and our ability to extract wisdom from what we're psychologically experiencing throughout our life experiences. When in balance, the brow chakra manifests its energy as emotional intelligence, perceptiveness, optimism, good memory, awareness, and having an overall calmed mind. When out of balance, this chakra expresses itself as narrow-mindedness, an inability to make plans for the future, a lack of imagination, obsession with psychic vision, spaciness, and even difficulty concentrating.

The seventh chakra, the last of the seven chakra model, sits atop the head and is aptly called the "crown chakra." Sahasrara in Sanskrit, the crown chakra is associated with the colors white or gold and also governs the pineal gland, parts of the hypothalamus, and parts of the immune system. Emotionally, this chakra is related to our sense of purpose and highest form of connection to the Divine. When in balance, the crown chakra manifests its energy as having a sense of unity with and love for the Divine, thoughtfulness, being open-minded, and the ability to receive and recognize divine guidance. When out of balance, this chakra expresses itself as spiritual addiction, confusion, dissociation from the physical body, sense of separation from the Divine, and difficulty believing in Divine help.

Now that we understand the fundamentals of each chakra, it is easy to see how something like a physical surgery that is brought on by trauma and ends in trauma can cause spiritual disruptions of all kinds. While being afforded the opportunity to sit and speak to a therapist is an important step towards cultivating healing, without understanding the missing piece that is our spiritually energetic anatomy, people can go to therapy and still feel as though something is lacking. Engaging in prayer as a means to promote healing, from the less clinical side of the spectrum, is also deeply helpful, but again, a clear understanding around what's been impacted can guide your prayer practices. Focusing on one area at a time in your prayer and even meditation can help you feel more balanced and less likely to jump to the conclusion that you aren't healing. Not understanding this anatomy and its subsequent impact on the power of your voice can have you jumping to conclusions that can potentially lead to unnecessary self-suppression or self-alienation.

Now with this full awareness of what each chakra is and its functioning, you can begin practicing discernment around your feelings and where your imbalance might be coming from. This gives you an opportunity to see whether your emotional responses are directly linked to the trauma of the surgery itself -- i.e.your digestive or nervous systems—or is it the impact of the surgery on the entirety of your life moving forward, pulling up deeper rooted issues that have gone unchecked until now. This is what I believe keeps most mothers stuck in painful cycles of fear with an inability to move forward—their bodies and emotions erupting in various manifestations of these spiritual imbalances. The fear of knowing you're not in a place that truly warrants a clinical diagnosis, but you're also not sure how you're going to make it through the next season of your life with so much in disarray, is enough to make anyone really, really pissed off. This is also particularly why I believe grounding contemplation in the Coping Self portion of the Indivisible Self model is a beautiful and practical bridge to prayer rehabilitation. You can feel supported whether or not you live in an environment where you have tons of help, resources, and support.

This astute attention to your feelings can help you hone in on what needs examining most. If you're like Diana and you find yourself practicing self-sabotage, then you know one of the reasons you're struggling to establish or develop a will that's in alignment with the Divine is because your sacral chakra is out of balance. Spending time journaling and reflecting on what's been surfacing, including what type of patterns you express when in relationship with others, can give you a healthy opportunity to observe and ask for Divine support to eventually release. I recommend an initial scan of all of the questions in each chakra set and then settling in with each chakra as it resonates. You might find you only need reflection with two or three at the moment, but the importance rests in knowing which needs the most care and attuning. Over time, you can always return to them should you ever feel the need to. Using the breath techniques, essential oils, and even affirmations from the Rest portion of the method will greatly support you as you work with this phase of the method. Let's begin the process of renewing your spiritual power!

~Root Chakra reflection questions (issues of perfectionism as a means of claiming/securing a role in the group)

1. How do I feel when I am not able to practice my motherhood in the way my mother, sister, or members of my tribe do?

2. What role does tradition play in my life when it comes to how I view family life? Do I feel isolated from doing things differently from everybody else?

3. Am I able to trust that doing things my own way will cultivate pleasant results? What is my fear teaching me in this moment?

~Sacral Chakra reflection questions (issues of perfectionism, establishing boundaries from fear of loss/alienation)

which is the power of connecting back to sexual purity, personal power, creativity and the possibility of a womb renewed also known as future births. Control and power dynamics, healing shame for giving away your power.

Here are questions for you to consider as you navigate the issues of power and your role in striking a balance with others during your recovery. Your financial contribution to your home life, the internal life and the speed with which you feel is necessary to heal.

1. How do I feel when I am not financially contributing to my home? How do my friends/social connections treat me when I am unable to fiscally contribute?

2. What role did money play in my upbringing? What did I learn about money and femininity? What did my mother, grandmother, great-grandmother think/feel/say/experience around the cultivation and earning of money?

3. Am I scared about losing all that I have cultivated creatively by taking rest?

~The Solar Plexus Chakra (issues of lack of perseverance, low self-esteem/ rebuilding personal self-esteem, self-confidence, endurance back to personal purpose and how to serve others)

1. How do I feel when my body needs more rest than my mind will allow?

2. How do I view my worthiness as a person when I am unable to complete certain tasks within a certain timeframe?

3. Am I afraid that if I cannot complete a project or plan something once I start, then stopping will ruin my efforts?

~The Heart Chakra (issues of Bitterness/ Resentment/ Judgmental)

1. How do I feel when I see other mothers resuming personal or professional activity faster than I?

2. How do I respond when other mothers share positive experiences in my presence?

3. What makes me feel like I should keep to myself? What in this season makes me believe or feel unloveable? open up vs. staying closed off, feeling loveable vs feeling loathsome.

~The Throat Chakra (issues of Timidity/Suppressing feelings/ Excessive talking/ Timing/)

1. How do I feel when I see other mothers resuming personal or professional activity faster than I?

2. How do I feel when I see other mothers express the joy or satisfaction in their own birthing experiences?

3. What do I fear will go wrong if I choose to trust my intuition as I rebuild this part of my life?

~The Brow Chakra (issues of confusion, unclear intuition, inability to use both logical and intuitive mind cohesively)

1. What makes me feel most confused about the path up ahead?

2. What prevents me from being able to make a plan or take actionable steps towards my healing?

3. What makes me feel discouraged in this season? What do I perceive as barriers to my progress?

~The Crown Chakra (issues of disconnection from source/ victimhood)

1. How do I feel when I go to pray?

2. Do I believe I can only access God's grace in one format?

3. What do I believe about the creator's love for motherhood?

How did it feel to go through each section? Were there chakras your intuition guided you to sit with more than others? Again, don't allow yourself to become overwhelmed, as this portion of reflection is here for you to revisit and work through at your leisure.

While the crown chakra wraps up the energetic system and how to pay attention to what feels most out of balance, the contemplation aspect is here to help you tie your journaling responses back to your prayer and meditation, if they've become too unfamiliar to lean on. As I mentioned in chapter one, when you go through experiences that trigger shock and grief, denying they've happened by clinging to gratitude can feel like the spiritually right thing to do. And while using gratitude to cultivate resilience makes sense, as many of us do, cultivating awareness of the spiritual body's needs postpartum is central to cultivating a rehabilitated connection to Source. The health and optimal wellness of our energetic anatomy, all the way up to the crown chakra, is fostered by this alignment and awareness. Using the Coping Self section of the Indivisible Self model I mentioned earlier, where you can look at each area of your daily postpartum responsibilities, I have crafted some questions using a contemplation point followed by an affirmation for rewiring the energy of the chakra so as to affirm the highest qualities of each energetic center and its relationship to these daily responsibilities. Again, these are directly from my own experiential wisdom using my faith-based approach, to help you explore any deeply ingrained beliefs keeping you from being able to move forward. If you are a member of another faith or simply like to stay open, I invite you to sit with each and explore how your spirit receives the information.

Contemplation point # 1

Leisure: Taking time to restore free-time and ease into the postpartum journey as I heal

Statement of Belief- "I am not weak, undisciplined, or lazy for taking time to be present in enjoying the laughter, development, and growth of my child(ren). I am a better mother when I am filled to the brim with peace and pleasantness."

Questions for Contemplation:

1. How did saying these words out loud make you feel?

2. Did you notice any visceral reactions in your body? Where?

3. Did you feel ashamed or like you needed permission for this statement to be true?

4. What in my living environment grants me the opportunity to elevate this space for play? Is there something in my environment or living condition that inhibits this? Is it within my control to change or adjust?

5. Where can I invite my spouse, partner, or friends to support me in this space for play?

Scriptural points of anchoring:

"A joyful heart is good medicine, but a crushed spirit dries up the bones." - Proverbs 17:22

"I do not concern myself with great matters or things too wonderful for me. But I have calmed and quieted myself. I am like a weaned child with its mother; like a weaned child I am content." - Psalm 131:1-2

"Dear friend, I pray that you may enjoy good health and all that may go well with you, even as your soul is getting along well." - 3 John 1:2

Contemplation point # 2

Stress Management: Evaluating how setting limits, establishing boundaries, and managing personal energy soothes during times of stress along the postpartum journey.

Statement of Belief- "I am not secretive, paranoid, or distrusting for establishing limits and boundaries around what I want to share about this place on my postpartum journey. I am free to determine how much of myself I can extend to others in this season. It is okay if others express displeasure or disdain around my choices.

Questions for Contemplation:

6. How did saying these words out loud make you feel?

7. Did you notice any visceral reactions in your body? Where?

8. Did you feel ashamed or like you needed permission for this statement to be true?

9. Who do you fear might judge you for not disclosing everything about your journey at the moment?

10. Who do you fear losing as you learn to navigate this part of your healing journey?

Scriptural point of anchoring:

"The Lord is my shepherd. I shall not want. He makes me to lay down in green pastures. He leads me beside still waters."- Psalms 23:1-2

"Be still and know, I am God."- Psalms 46:10

"And the effect of righteousness will be peace, and the result of righteousness, quietness and trust forever."- Isaiah 32:17

"Turn my eyes away from worthless things; preserve my life according to your word." - Psalms 119: 50

"The Lord is my light and my salvation, whom shall I fear? The Lord is the stronghold of my life; of whom shall I be afraid?"- Psalm 27:1

"My comfort in suffering is this: your promise preserves my life."- Psalms 119:50

Contemplation point # 3

Self-worth: Taking time to affirm who you are in this season of the postpartum journey and that the stage you are in matters, even if you are used to being a strong or resilient person but do not feel such or cannot be at the moment. Your ability to recognize all your positive qualities and how they can be appropriately transferred/used during this season to help you grow as a mother.

Statement of Belief- "I am not dwelling in the fragility of my c-section trauma. I am consciously making every effort to rebuild my mind, body, and spirit at a pace that neither frustrates nor rushes me. My progress indicates I am concerned and committed to growth and personal development in this season.

Questions for Contemplation:

11. How did saying these words out loud make you feel?

12. Did you notice any visceral reactions in your body? Where?

13. Did you feel ashamed or like you needed permission for this statement to be true?

14. Do you feel there is a way you should look and sound while in this stage of your journey?

15. How do you feel about your flaws showing up right now? Is there someone in your immediate environment who makes it difficult for you to let your flaws be seen? How can you begin to engage them in conversation to understand what support you currently need?

Scriptural point of anchoring:

"I praise you, for I am fearfully and wonderfully made. Wonderful are your works; my soul knows it very well." -Psalms 139:14

"But He said to me, 'My grace is sufficient for you, for my power is made perfect in weakness.'"- 2 Corinthians 12:9

Contemplation point # 4

Realistic Beliefs: Your ability to recognize your current reality for what it is. Your ability to understand the role of motherhood from a personal, cultural, and societal perspective. Your ability to discern technologically-influenced reality from personal reality.

Statement of Belief- "I am not tied or restricted to patterns, expectations, or influences pushed via social media or other media outlets. I recognize and accept how my culture, level of education, religious/spiritual beliefs, and the environment I live in influences my postpartum journey.

Questions for Contemplation:

16. How did saying these words out loud make you feel?

17. Did you notice any visceral reactions in your body? Where?

18. Did you feel ashamed or like you needed permission for this statement to be true?

19. Do you feel social media or other media outlets are the true

source of authority for how you make personal decisions?

20. How do you feel when you are unable to live out your motherhood the way it is being marketed through these various mediums? What keeps you stuck in this feeling?

Scriptural point of anchoring:

"I praise you, for I am fearfully and wonderfully made. Wonderful are your works; my soul knows it very well." -Psalms 139:14

"But He said to me, 'My grace is sufficient for you, for my power is made perfect in weakness.'"- 2 Corinthians 12:9

Chapter 9

Speaking Your Way Forward

———

January 2021 was on its way and so was the opportunity to try my hand, once again, at the soup that sets the tone for freedom in my home. The end of the year and the beginning of a new one often came in waves after my son's birth, but for the first time since his birth, despite the unexpectedness of being in a pandemic, I felt excited to make the soup. Trusting the practice I had put into every aspect of the method up until this point, I felt a certain groundedness moving forward that hadn't been present before. Matched with a sense of bubbling urgency, I set out to grocery shop a little more intentionally than years prior. As the matriarch of my own home, picking out the perfect pumpkin and every single ingredient needed for the beloved freedom soup was my responsibility. But it also gave me a chance to notice just how full-circle I had come through all the Januarys since that first one of the birth. This particular January, I finally felt grounded, paced, and nourished enough to not be scared of moving through this anniversary mentally, physically, emotionally, and yes, spiritually. I had finally reached a place where I felt my true freedom.

While I chopped fresh carrots, minced fresh garlic, and began seasoning fresh pieces of beef, I smiled to myself. I reflected on how I'd found freedom through the deeply engaging conversations I'd had with fellow mothers. I smiled at all the ways I had chosen to initiate healing. I smiled at the deep inner knowing that the path to healing I had aligned myself with wasn't easy, but it felt soul deep. This path I have chosen to share with you didn't magically erase the daily reminders of a surgery I didn't need or the lingering wonder around how differently things could have gone had I not had it, but it managed to support a heart that had been cracked wide open, cracked wide open with rage, betrayal, sadness and disappointment. This path pointed me in the direction of true healing and gave me an ability to reclaim my voice. I no longer found myself stuck in a place of woundedness or resentment, but now lived in a place of exploration of how this newly discovered freedom could yield a more loving postpartum journey.

In letting go of all the fear, shame, angst, and feelings of defeat I had felt since the day I had to surrender to the power struggle brought on by my practitioner, I learned to stretch, sway, bend, empty out, lay still and accept transformation—and these practices gave me freedom. I learned to accept that I might never cross paths with my former practitioner and that forgiving her for what her stubbornness cost me was never truly the point as I had originally thought. In fact, I learned through these years, and each season of remembrance, that this was really about teaching me how to turn inwards and grant myself the permission to initiate healing in the way I wanted and desperately needed. While the actions taken by my practitioner were some that should have been punished, I rectify it all by taking back my spiritual power in being able to talk about it, openly and honestly. I take back my power by living in freedom as I heal.

There is no easy way to move forward, nor is there any magic wand that can be waved to erase the pain that c-section birth trauma causes. But through reading these very personal accounts and experiences, there is a way to feel less alone in your experience of putting the pieces back together and reclaiming a much brighter and more restored postpartum journey. The Whole Mother Method can help us challenge the notion that there is no way to feel sorrowful, angry, and downright heartbroken without being typecast as automatically having a mental health issue. Understanding how healing can happen when we incorporate the mind, body, and spirit can help us steer our postpartum healing in a way that makes us feel more empowered, less ashamed, and less categorized. While we know mental illness can be triggered by trauma, we also know being of sound mind can start from a healed body and repurposed spiritual wind. This doesn't happen overnight or without the proper resources. Writing this love-letter of sorts to you was with this reality in mind.

As we go our separate ways, I leave these affirmations as a form of blessing and my prayer is you carry these truths in your spirit, with you always—

- Becoming a Mother is an act of divinity—c-section birth trauma doesn't get to steal the power from that.

- You are destined for more (peace, grace, beauty, love, self-understanding)— c-section birth trauma can't stop you from receiving it all.

- Your story matters—c-section birth trauma doesn't silence your voice.

Appendix

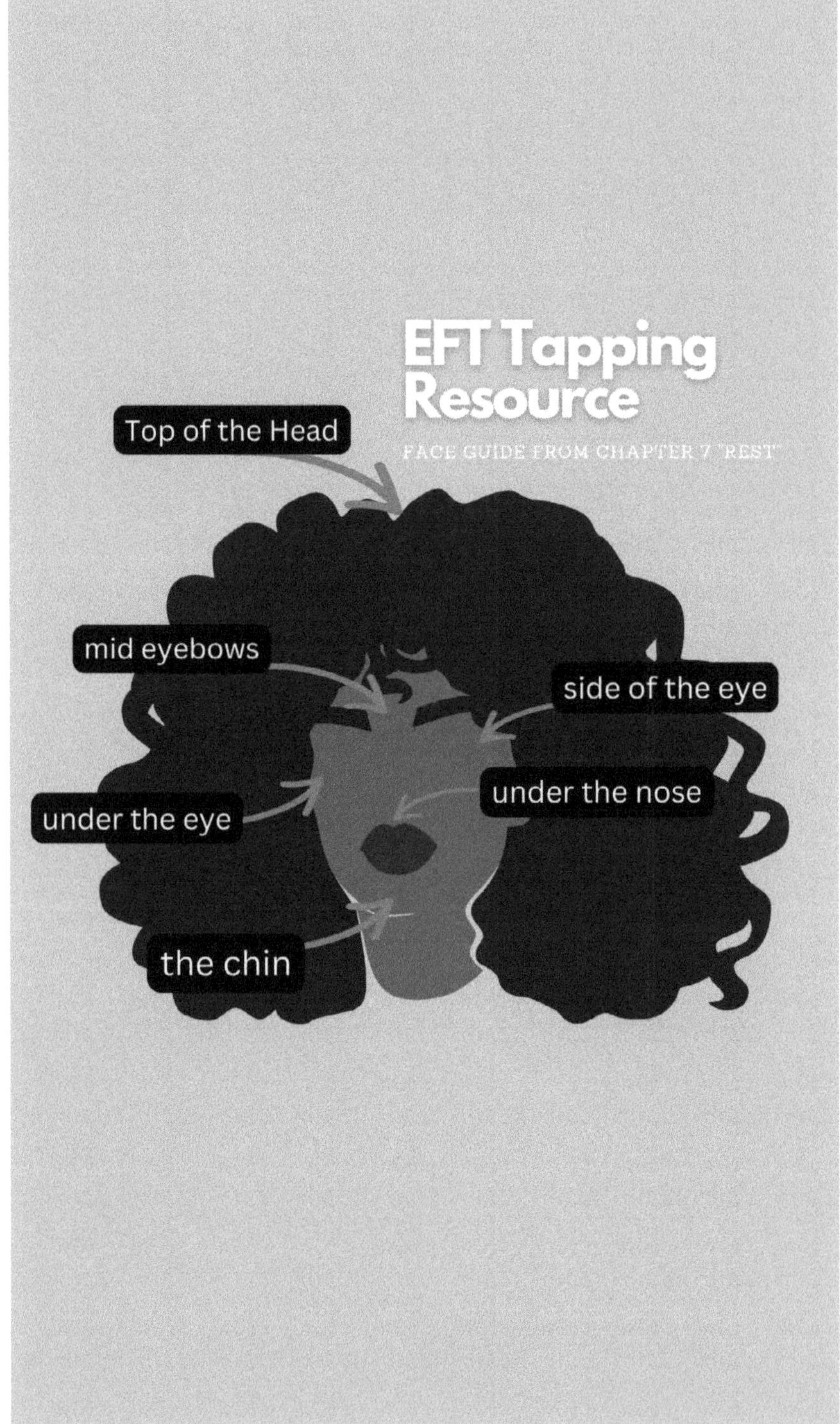

EFT Tapping
Resource
FACE GUIDE FROM CHAPTER 7 "REST"
Top of the Head
mid eyebows
side of the eye
under the nose
under the eye
the chin

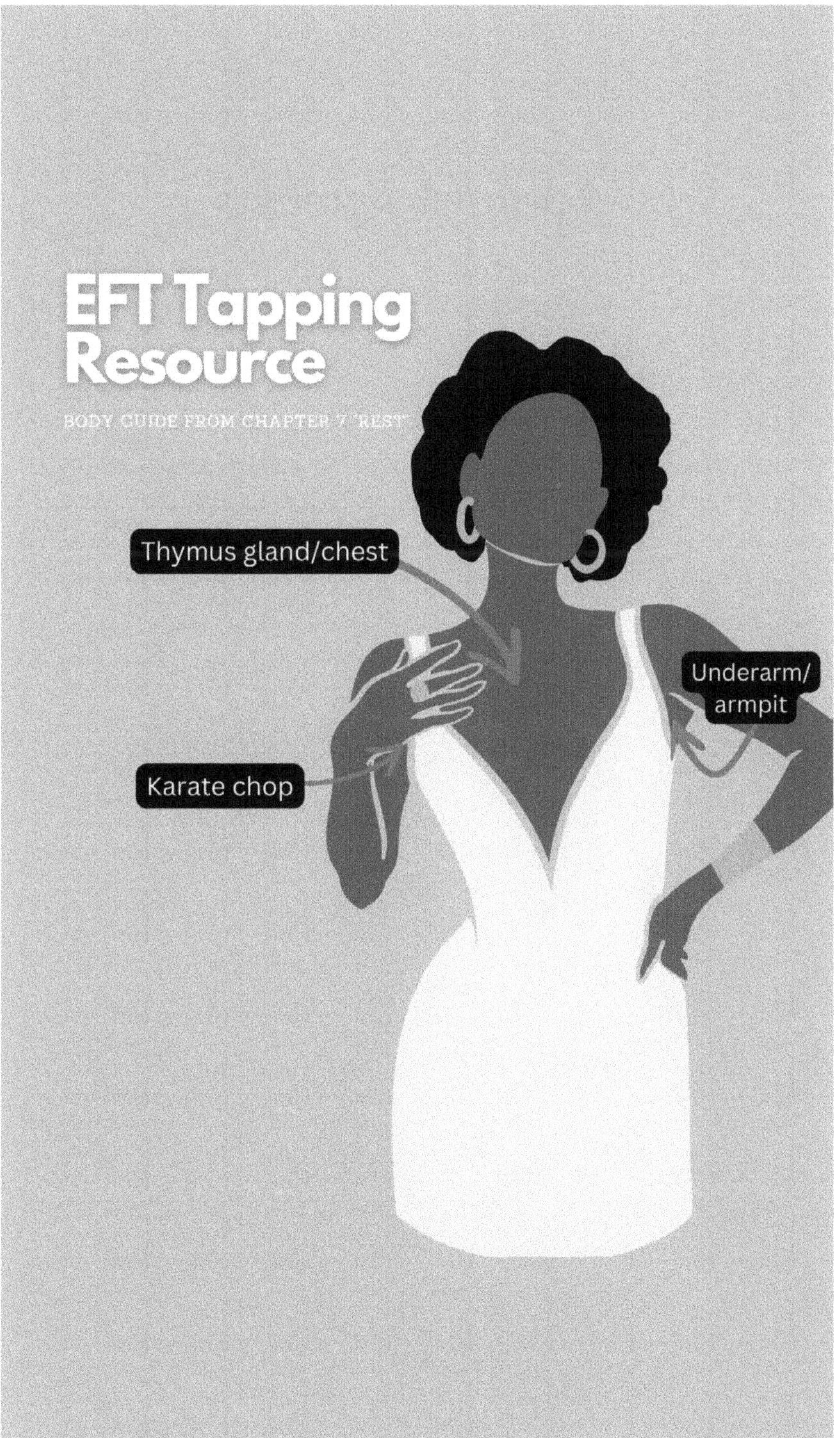
EFT Tapping
Resource
BODY GUIDE FROM CHAPTER 7 "REST"
Thymus gland/chest
Underarm/
armpit
Karate chop

Acknowledgments

Writing this book was an experience that could not have been possible without God's unyielding love and help, so to Him I say thank you, first and foremost. I would like to thank my husband for listening to me read draft after draft, despite being brought down such a painful memory lane at times. My children for their patience and encouragement because they know how important it is for "mommy to teach the people through her storytelling." I'd like to thank KN Literary and my editor Katie Booth for walking with me through the sometimes daunting process of editing. Your feedback and dedication, Katie, was instrumental in making this work more than just my story, but a guide for others to lean on and learn from. Thank you to the nurses who were like guardian angels at a time I needed them most. And finally, thank you to you, the reader, for allowing this book to be a source of support.

Notes

Chapter One

1 Soderquist, J., Wijma, K., & Wijma, B. Traumatic Stress after Childbirth: The Role of Obstetric Variables. Journal of Psychosomatic Obstetrics & Gynecology, (2002) 23(1), 31–39.

2 Kim Thomas, "What is Birth Trauma?" The Birth Trauma Association, 2018, https://birthtraumaassociation.org.uk/for-parents/what-is-birth-trauma.

3 Pablo Noriega, Bach Flower Essences and Chinese Medicine(Healing Arts Press, 2016).

4 Cyndi Dale, The Subtle Body: An Encyclopedia of Your Energetic Anatomy, (Sounds True, 2009)

Chapter Four

5 American Psychological Association. (2021) Apology to people of color for APA's role in promoting, perpetuating, and failing to challenge racism, racial discrimination, and human hierarchy in U. S. https://www.apa.org/about/policy/racism-apology

6 Stengler, Mark, et al. "Aromatherapy Basics." Prescription for Natural Cures: A Self-Care Guide for Treating Health Problems with Natural Remedies Including Diet, Nutrition, Supplements, and Other Holistic Methods, Turner Publishing Company, Nashville, TN, 2016, pp. 773–773.

Chapter Six

7 Church D, Stapleton P, Vasudevan A, O'Keefe T. Clinical EFT as an evidence-based practice for the treatment of psychological and physiological conditions: A systematic review. Front Psychol. 2022 Nov 10;13:951451. doi: 10.3389/fpsyg.2022.951451. PMID: 36438382; PMCID: PMC9692186.

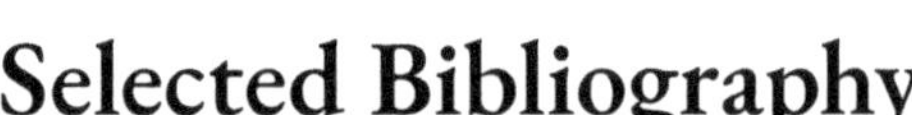

Selected Bibliography

"Knowledge, attitudes, and practices regarding gemstone therapeutics in a selected adult population in Pakistan." National Institute of Mental Health, U.S. Department of Health and Human Services, https://www.ncbi.nlm.nih.gov/pmc/articles/PMC2739841. Date accessed. 15 May 2022

"Post-Traumatic Stress Disorder." National Institute of Mental Health, U.S. Department of Health and Human Services, https://www.nimh.nih.gov/health/topics/post-traumatic-stress-disorder-ptsd. Date accessed. 15, May 2022.

A., Van der Kolk Bessel. The Body Keeps the Score: Mind, Brain and Body in the Transformation of Trauma. Penguin Books, 2015.

Beers, Mark H., editor. The Merck Manual of Medical Information. Merck Publications, 1997.

Ivey, Allen E., and Mary Bradford Ivey. Intentional Interviewing and Counseling: Facilitating Client Development in a Multicultural Society. Braille Jymico Inc., 2003.

Lasater, Judith Hanson. Relax and Renew Restful Yoga for Stressful Times. Shambhala, 2016.

Minetor, Randi. Essential Oils of the Bible: Connecting God's Word to Natural Healing, Althea Press, Berkeley, CA, 2016.

Myss, Caroline M. Anatomy of the Spirit the Seven Stages of Power and Healing. Harmony Books, 2017.

Noriega, Pablo, and Loey Colebeck. Bach Flower Essences and Chinese Medicine. Healing Arts Press, 2016.

S., Iyenger B K. Light on Yoga. Schocken Books, 1966.

SERRALLACH, DR OSCAR. The Postnatal Depletion Cure, Grand Central Life & Style, New York, NY, 2018.

Shea, Bridgette. Handbook of Chinese Medicine and Ayurveda: An Integrated Practice of Ancient Healing Traditions, Healing Arts Press, Rochester, VT, 2018.

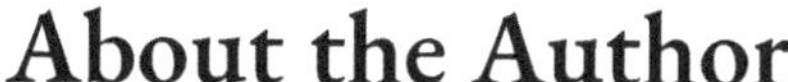

About the Author

———

Laura Eustache Zamor, BCDN, CHHP, believes the health of a mother directly impacts the health and strength of her family, and society at large. However, whole person wellness can only occur when a mother is given the knowledge and wherewithal to make decisions that support her overall empowerment. Dr. Zamor's work then, is dedicated to helping mothers, and their families, understand the connection between the mind, body, and spirit when it comes to achieving this overall health and empowerment. Through advocacy around sharing the sometimes more undiscussed realities of motherhood, her intention is to help mothers recover pieces of themselves lost through traumatic experiences for a more restorative postpartum journey.

Dr. Zamor is a Board Certified Doctor of Naturopathy, Certified Holistic Health Practitioner, and traditional Herbalist who holds a Masters of Education in Counseling & School Counseling. Having held positions in Student Affairs to School Counseling, Dr. Zamor is the author of a previous work, "The Audacity to Finish," and the producer/host of the three season podcast, "#thebeautifulstruggle." Previously, her work and advocacy for owning one's personal narrative has been presented through platforms such as the former Book Expo's Ingram stage and local news media such as "BronxNet." Dr. Zamor is a featured contributor on the weekly community radio show, "Causerie Holistik" for RadioAfrica1804.com where she discusses, in Haitian Kreyol, all things holistic health and wellness. She is the owner of Kay Grann Apothecary®, an herbal apothecary providing handcrafted blends, tinctures, and signature tea for emotional as well as digestive wellness. She lives, writes, and teaches in NYC with her husband and two children.